PRAISE FOR FOOD OVER MEDICINE

"Very few people, and even very few doctors, really understand how powerful nutrition can be in preventing and in treating most of the illnesses that afflict us today. *Food Over Medicine* is an outstanding resource for anyone wanting to maximize their health and minimize their dependence on western medicine."

—JOHN ROBBINS,
author of *No Happy Cows* and *Diet for a New America*

"*Food Over Medicine* explains nutrition in an original, highly compelling way. A totally digestible, accessible approach to learning how to maintain or regain your health."

—RORY FREEDMAN, author of *Skinny Bitch*

"Reading *Food Over Medicine* is like having nutrition explained to you in a no-nonsense way by a dear friend. This is not some dry textbook; it's a jargon-free conversation—one that will change your life!" —LINDSAY S. NIXON,
author of the bestselling Happy Herbivore
cookbook series

"*Food Over Medicine* is brimming with useful information that is both detailed and yet easy to understand. The question-and-answer format is very effective with excellent points. It's the sort of book that everyone who cares about their health should read."

—LEE FULKERSON, director of *Forks Over Knives*

"*Food Over Medicine* is a must for anyone remotely concerned about health. It is incredibly funny, totally engaging, and promotes a diet that just happens to be the best for the planet."

—ED BEGLEY JR., actor and environmental activist

"Reading *Food Over Medicine* could be the best health insurance you ever had. This no-nonsense approach to solid health information may save your life!" —HOWARD F. LYMAN, author of *Mad Cowboy* and *No More Bull!*

"*Food Over Medicine* is an excellent book that reveals the truth that health is more about dietary choices and plant-based nutrition than about doctors, diagnostic tests, surgeries, procedures, and medications. The book is easy-to-read, entertaining, and humorous. But, above all else, it is incredibly informative, enlightening, inspiring, and self-empowering. It will open your eyes. It will encourage you to take charge of your life."
—DR. WALTER R. JACOBSEN, author of *Forgive to Win!*

"*Food Over Medicine* cuts through every nutrition-related controversy to give you the information you need for a lifetime of health and trim weight." —JANICE STANGER, PH.D., author of *The Perfect Formula Diet*

FOOD
OVER
MEDICINE

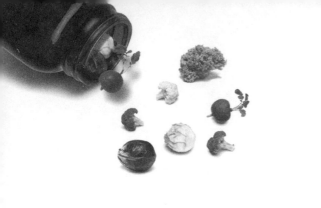

FOOD
OVER
MEDICINE

THE CONVERSATION
THAT COULD SAVE YOUR LIFE

PAMELA A. POPPER PH.D., N.D. and GLEN MERZER

BENBELLA BOOKS, INC.
DALLAS, TEXAS

BenBella

BenBella Books, Inc.
10300 Central Expressway, Suite #530
Dallas, TX 75231
www.benbellabooks.com
Send feedback to feedback@benbellabooks.com

Printed in the United States of America
10 9 8 7 6 5 4 3 2 1
Library of Congress Cataloging-in-Publication Data is available for this title.
Popper, Pamela.
  Food over medicine : the conversation that could save your life / by Pamela A. Popper, Ph.D., N.D., and Glen Merzer.
      pages cm
  Includes bibliographical references and index.
  ISBN 978-1-937856-80-9 (trade cloth : alk. paper) -- ISBN 978-1-937856-57-1 (e-book) 1. Nutritionally induced diseases--Popular works. 2. Diet in disease--Popular works. 3. Food habits--Popular works. 4. Health behavior--Popular works. I. Merzer, Glen. II. Title.
  RA645.N87P663 2013
  616.3'9--dc23
2013004503

Editing by Erin Kelley
Copy Editing by Lisa Miller
Proofreading by Chris Gage and Michael Fedison
Text design and composition by Elyse Strongin, Neuwirth & Associates, Inc.
Cover photography by Robert Merrill
Food Photographs by Robert Metzger
Printed by Bang Printing

Distributed by Perseus Distribution
To place orders through Perseus Distribution:
Tel: 800-343-4499
Fax: 800-351-5073
E-mail: orderentry@perseusbooks.com
www.perseusdistribution.com

Significant discounts for bulk sales are available. Please contact Glenn Yeffeth at glenn@benbellabooks.com or (214) 750-3628.

This book is dedicated to all of the people who have listened to my lectures, read my books, joined the Wellness Forum, improved their health, and shared their stories during the last sixteen years. You have all inspired me to continue to tell the truth about diet, health, and medicine.

And also to the great pioneers who have influenced my work—Dr. John McDougall, Dr. T. Colin Campbell, Dr. Caldwell Esselstyn, Dr. Neal Barnard, Dr. Alan Goldhamer, Dr. Doug Lisle, Dr. Peter Breggin, William Lessler, Dr. Ralph Moss, and many other colleagues from whom I continue to learn every day.

Last but not least, to my parents who taught me that anything is possible with hard work and persistence.

—*Pamela A. Popper*

CONTENTS

ACKNOWLEDGMENTS

We would like to express our gratitude to Amanda Crichton, who helped in more ways that we can count, to Jill Hiller, for her assistance with graphics, and to Nicole Swartz for her assistance in archiving the research for this book. Thanks also to Kelly Sherman, Gary Morse, Del Sroufe, and Cindy Beebe, who help to run The Wellness Forum, often without Pam, which allows for projects like this book.

Thank you to Chef Del for contributing many of his delicious recipes.

Thank you also to Robert Merrill and Robert Metzger for the photography, and to Nicole Schlosser and Erin Kelley for their superb editorial assistance. We appreciate as well the input of Jana Germano, David Nemtzow, John Tanner, and Dr. Pamela Russo.

And our most heartfelt thanks go to the many Wellness Forum members: "Darcy," Maureen Yatwa, Jill Collett, Barry and Elisabeth Small, Patty Yeager, "Martin," Ellen Seigel, Cat Timmons, Janet Triner, Larry Nicol, and, once again, the incomparable Wellness Forum Chef Del Sroufe for sharing their very personal stories so that others can learn from them and regain their health.

INTRODUCTION

. . . .

Nutrition must rank near the top of subjects that are vitally important to the human experience, and yet are still poorly understood. Textbooks on the subject tend to be dry, intended to be read only by professionals in the field, such as nutritionists and dietitians. Popular books that address the subject generally take the form of diet books, designed to hawk the latest weight-loss fad and skew all research in favor of the diet being sold. The news offers us only snippets of nutritional information, devoid of context and misinterpreted, leaving millions of Americans believing that fish oil will protect them from heart attacks, that chocolate holds the key to longevity, or that low-fat ice cream is a health food. And so they continue to eat themselves into an early grave.

Furthermore, even those who eat a sound diet may still end up experiencing poor health as a result of interaction with the medical system. There is little evidence to support the use of many of the tests, drugs, supplements, and procedures commonly recommended by a majority of health care practitioners. Most medical professionals do not make full and honest disclosures about the minimal (or nonexistent) benefits of these medical interventions, or about their risks and side effects.

Sorting out the confusion perpetuated by the barrage of conflicting information on the topic takes more time and expertise than the average person has. We may not all be up for reading a scientific textbook, but on a matter as important as our own health, we're all up for a good talk. So we thought we'd take a shot at bringing these subjects to life through conversation.

We hope you'll like it, and we hope you'll walk away with an understanding that will improve your health.

Pam Popper

Glen Merzer

DEEP-FRIED BUTTER ON A STICK AND OTHER ATROCITIES

. . . .

GLEN MERZER: Pam, how would you characterize the overall state of the health of Americans as a population? How sick are we?

PAM POPPER: Very sick and very overweight. It's far worse than most people believe.

GM: But aren't we living longer than before?

PP: We're not living longer in good health; we're living fractionally longer with diseases that compromise our quality of life and that cost us a fortune. We're living longer with diseases like diabetes and Alzheimer's, which are both seeing explosive growth in the number of diagnoses. And, in fact, we're not living that long at all; we're around thirty-sixth among nations on the longevity charts, tied with our very poor neighbor Cuba. We're in a health crisis. We spend more money by far than any other nation on health yet we have miserable health outcomes. Some people don't perceive it that way. We have to change their minds.

GM: What's making Americans so sick?

PP: Our food. And I say that for two reasons: One, we have excellent data on populations with lower disease rates and we know that their eating patterns are different than ours. Two, we have excellent data on the rare physicians who use diet as an intervention tool, showing that when people adopt the right diet, they often eat their way out of their diseases. Diet is clearly the problem.

GM: Has a nation ever existed that is fatter than America today?

PP: Never in recorded history have we seen such obesity. We've set the record. And it's going to be tough to beat.

GM: There's been a lot of attention paid to obesity recently. Do you see any signs of improvement?

PP: It's getting worse, unfortunately. When I was doing research for *Forks Over Knives*, I was looking at obesity statistics; the statement was made in the film that 40 percent of Americans are obese. If you take a look at the website of the Centers for Disease Control, the party line is that a third of the country is obese. Well, if you take a look at how we categorize obesity and overweight conditions in our country based on body mass index charts, we're basically saying 21 to 24 percent is normal, 25 to 29 percent is overweight, 30 percent and higher is obese, and 40 percent and higher means you're morbidly obese. Well in India, 21 to 24 is overweight, not normal.[1] This is also the approach in Canada[2] and many other countries. If you pick up the population of the United States and plop it down in the middle of India and other countries with higher standards than ours, our obesity rate would approach 60 percent.

GM: So there's a potential way out of the crisis. Just lower our standards a little more. Define "overweight" as "twice as fat as an obese Indian."

PP: It's almost unbelievable. No other population has ever had such unlimited access to so many bad foods to become this over-weight. And no population has ever been as misled as ours by a perverse system of incentives in food manufacturing, the advertising industry, and the medical field. So we've eaten ourselves into the dubious distinction of being the fattest population in re-corded history; now we've got to figure out how we're going to teach more than three hundred million people to eat their way out of this terrible state.

GM: I heard a report on NPR about the healthiest, fittest, and leanest state in America: Colorado.[3] The reporter went on about all the joggers, the bike paths in Boulder, and the skiing in Aspen. Then he actually said, "In fitness-crazy Colorado, the obesity rate is only 21 percent."[4]

PP: So that's only about a million people.

GM: Yup. That's our skinniest population. That's as good as it gets. And, credit where credit is due, only one in four children in Colo-rado is overweight or obese.

I've noticed that people just assume that it's normal to gain weight as you age. Friends who were 160 pounds in college hit middle age and they're 200 pounds. Is there any reason why a fifty-year-old should weigh more than he did when he was twenty or twenty-five?

PP: The only reason why a fifty-year-old would weigh more than he did when he was twenty or twenty-five is that his diet and lifestyle finally caught up with him. Youth will overcome a great number of indiscretions. That's why people tend to get cancer a little later in life; it takes that long for the dietary habits to catch up. It's simply diet and lifestyle habits catching up, with the major habit being exercise, or lack thereof. I'm fifty-six years old and the vast majority of people my age are not doing the right amount of exercise; some of them don't exercise at all. Gaining weight is not a normal function of aging. There's no reason why you can't stay lean and physically active into your nineties and be healthy.

GM: What would you say are the leading causes of our unmatched record of obesity?

PP: First, there is an overall confusion about food and the way that people are taught to eat from a very early age. We have strange ideas about food in this country. One is the idea that moderation is the key to success, that you can eat almost anything you want as long as you eat it in moderation.

GM: I hear that a lot, though no one ever says it about hemlock.

PP: I attended a wedding last night and food was the topic of the table. I wasn't eating 90 percent of what they served, and the guy next to me said, "Everything in moderation is okay, so I'm just going to have a little bit of this stuff." Well, it was a little bit of a bunch of horrible things that added up to probably 2,500 calories, 2,000 of them from fat. You know, that's not moderation—that's a diet that kills people. We have a lot of misbegotten ideas about food, many of which come from the government, national health organizations like the Academy of Nutrition and Dietetics, and other professional groups.

Another part of it is the availability of rich, inexpensive food. If you go back several hundred years, you used to have the wealthy and poor eating vastly different diets. The wealthy ate rich food with lots of calories, with the result often being health and weight problems. The poor peasants couldn't afford rich food so they lived on potatoes and vegetables for most of the year. A few times a year they'd have a festival and roast a pig, but then it was back to vegetables and potatoes. The fact that they didn't have the economic wherewithal to eat as the wealthy ate was protective for them; it kept them leaner and healthier than the wealthy. Today, most Americans can afford to eat meat and animal foods—things that used to be reserved for the wealthy. They're eating all of this calorie-dense animal food and processed and packaged food, day in and day out. And it's often a lot easier and sometimes cheaper in the inner city to find Kentucky Fried Chicken or McDonald's than fresh produce, so many people find themselves almost trapped into obesity. The cost of many animal foods is effectively kept low by federal farm subsidies, so our tax dollars are being used to skew our diet in the direction of the very foods that make us sick and obese.

When you eat this calorie-dense food, as Doug Lisle says in the movie *Forks Over Knives*, "People have to overeat just to be satisfied." If I'm going to try to fill my belly with cheese and potato chips, I've got to eat four thousand calories of it to accomplish that goal. You can't eat those foods without becoming overweight because you're forced to overconsume from a caloric standpoint. That's why we have an obesity epidemic in this country. Then you add to it the sedentary lifestyle of most people, and it's no wonder we're gaining weight at an alarming rate.

GM: Are you forced to overeat those foods to feel full because they're deficient in fiber?

PP: Yes. There are two mechanisms by which people experience what we call satiety: stretch receptors and nutrient receptors. Stretch receptors in the stomach tell you that the bulk of the food that you ate is sufficient, and that's where fiber is really helpful; if you eat a bowl of lentils and rice with fourteen grams of fiber, you're going to feel full. In fact, you couldn't overeat it because if you tried to eat four bowls of it, you'd explode. On the other hand, if I'm eating calorie-dense, fiber-deficient food (such as a turkey sandwich and potato chips), in order to activate those stretch receptors, I've got to eat an enormous amount of calories. We only feel satiety when the stretch receptors and the nutrient receptors in our stomach tell us that we've had enough bulk of food and calorie concentration. So with these calorie-dense, nutrient-deficient, and fiber-deficient foods, in order to activate those stretch receptors, you've got to eat a gargantuan quantity of calories to accomplish that goal, sometimes thousands of calories in a single meal. When you take into consideration that an average adult may need only two thousand calories per day, you can see the problem. It's easy to consume half of this in one meal.

GM: Tell me about the nutrient receptors. How do they work?

PP: They tell you if the calorie density of the food is adequate. That becomes important because just as you can overeat from a caloric standpoint by eating the standard American diet with animal foods and processed foods, you can also undereat by structuring a plant-based diet the wrong way. I see this often with people coming into our classes, people who have seen various movies or read articles and decided, "I'm going to eat a lot of fruits and vegetables. In fact, I'm going to structure my entire diet around fruits and vegetables." So they eat fruit for breakfast, have a big salad for lunch, and a big salad for dinner. After about three days of that, they're ready to chew their desk up at the office and can't sleep at night from the rumbling stomach. They're uncomfortable all the time and have a nagging hunger. Even when their stomachs are full of a pound and a half of vegetables, they have this nagging feeling of needing more food. Why? If I eat a pound and a half of vegetables, my stomach is going to be full from a bulk standpoint, but my nutrient receptors are going to say, "One hundred fifty calories? Gosh, I don't know if we can keep this human operating for another four hours on 150 calories!" I may be full from a fiber standpoint, but I'm not doing well based on my body's perception of the calorie density of the food. So we advise people to include a lot of grains and legumes and potatoes in their diet because they add calorie density to the meals without adding lots of fat and too many calories. Nature's perfect plan for humans.

GM: So that's the argument for having starch as a staple of the diet?

PP: Well, you have to. If you don't, here's what happens to people who try to live on fruits and vegetables. They go through what I call the "honeymoon period," when they benefit from what they take out of the diet. When they remove animal and junk foods from their diet, they feel great. They lose weight, their skin clears up, their headaches go away, and they say, "Boy, this is the greatest thing since right turn on a red light." However, within a few weeks they start to feel fatigued because the effect of the calorie deficiency sets in.

What a lot of people will do then is to start adding dried fruits, nuts, or oils to their diet. There are a lot of unhealthful plant-based options people choose to increase the calorie count. Over time, those people will develop health issues, generally speaking, as much as the meat eaters will. A plant-based diet won't work effectively if you don't do it right. And just eating fruits and vegetables is one of the ways that people can mess it up for themselves and a major reason why people revert to their old eating patterns. Then they say, "Well, this diet must not work. I have to go back to what I was doing before. It may not have been the best thing based on what I read in so-and-so's book, but at least I was able to stay awake all day and I was able to sleep at night because my stomach wasn't rumbling."

GM: The word "starch" seems to have a lousy public relations guy. People always have terrible things to say about starch. Dieters say that they're trying to avoid starchy foods and that they gain weight whenever they eat starch. What's the deal here? How can the type of food that actually helps people lose weight and stay healthy have such a bad reputation?

PP: That's because there are different sorts of foods that get labeled as "starch," and because starch often travels in bad company. In other words, people slather sour cream on their baked potato or olive oil on their pasta or pesto on their rice. You walk into a Mexican restaurant and instead of having the healthy starch of beans and rice, you order refried beans with lard inside a burrito with cheese in it—a 1,500-calorie, fat-laden Mexican dish.

Let's posit a hierarchy of starch. The healthiest starch comes from whole, unprocessed foods, such as whole grains, potatoes, sweet potatoes, yams, corn, and so forth. The next healthiest but suboptimal starch comes from broken grains, also known as flours. Whole wheat bread, for example, is denser and more caloric than wheat berries in their original form, but whole wheat flour itself is not inherently fatty or unhealthy. If you're trying to lose weight, staying away from broken grains is probably a good idea because broken grains are more concentrated in calories and generally don't have as much fiber as whole grains, so they're absorbed quickly in the system. The worst starch comes in refined foods and is combined with fats and sugars in products like muffins and cake. These starchy foods will put weight on you fast, but it's largely because of the added fats and sugars. People are misunderstanding the nature and importance of starch if the word conjures in their minds the image of donuts. It should conjure the image of yams and corn and rice.

GM: So it's simplistic and misleading to say that carbs are fattening?

PP: When people tell me carbohydrates are fattening, I tell them, "You know, two billion Asians never got that memo."

GM: What are the foods you recommend that have sufficient calorie density that make you feel full? What are the best foods to make the staples of your diet?

PP: Whole grains, legumes, and starchy vegetables. More broadly, I tell people to make the staples of their diet the four food groups, which are whole grains, legumes, fruits, and vegetables. We have our own little pyramid that we use here at The Wellness Forum. Beans, rice, corn, and potatoes are at the bottom of the pyramid. Then steamed and raw vegetables and big salads come next, with fruits after that. Whole grains, or premade whole grain foods like cereals and breads, are all right to eat. Everything else is either optional or a condiment.

As for high-fat plant foods—nuts, seeds, avocados, olives—use them occasionally or when they're part of a recipe, but don't overdo it; these foods are calorie-dense and full of fat. No oils, get rid of the dairy, and then, very importantly, you need to differentiate between food and a treat. I don't think you can get through to people by telling a twenty-five-year-old that she can't have

9

another cookie or a piece of cake for the rest of her life. Where you can gain some traction is to say, "Look, birthday parties are a good time for cake, Christmas morning is a good time for cookies, and Valentine's Day is a good time for chocolate, but you don't need to be eating that stuff all the time." People end up in my office because they're treating themselves several times a day.

GM: I had obese relatives who are gone now, my aunt and uncle. When I told them at the age of seventeen that I had gone vegetarian, they became terribly concerned that I wouldn't get enough protein. They weren't tall and must have weighed more than two hundred pounds each. Their kids were overweight, but they were worried about *me*. Usually they were on one diet or another, but they would make an exception for cake and ice cream on special occasions. And the special occasions were their birthdays, their kids' birthdays, their kids' spouses' birthdays, anniversaries, holidays, Earth Day, National Organ Donor Awareness Week ... the list went on and on.

PP: Right. You really have to put some common sense into this. My sister turned fifty a couple of years ago, which is a pretty big deal. We had cake and champagne, but there was no cake and champagne the next day or the next day or the next day. These have to be occasional treats; I tell people to make them situational. In other words, don't keep this stuff around the house because they'll call your name from the kitchen. I have no trouble staying away from cheese and animal food. But sweets, that's a different story; they're not as easy to resist. Not having any around is the easiest way to avoid them. If I want something sweet to eat after I get off work at ten o'clock, I've got bananas, plums, oranges, some apples, and some strawberries in my house. That's it. If I want anything else, I have to get in the car and go out and get it, something I'm not going to do at ten o'clock at night. It's a much better plan than standing in the kitchen saying, "Huh, I could have soy ice cream or I could have some cookies or I could have a banana or an apple." That's a choice that puts me in a position to have to use willpower.

GM: I used to have a sweet tooth. From the time I was a kid, I would always have cookies and cake and ice cream in the evening. Even when I became concerned about health as a teenager and became first a vegetarian and then, close to twenty years later, a vegan, I would still have a few vegan cookies in the evening. In the summer, I would follow that up with some soy ice cream. And then it turned out that my cholesterol kept creeping up on what I thought was an excellent diet. It was embarrassing. I had already coauthored with Howard Lyman two books on diet, and yet my cholesterol was 212 and my triglycerides were 203. My doctor recommended that I consider taking a statin drug to lower my cholesterol, which would have been really embarrassing. Now, I have bad genes. There have been a lot of heart attacks in my family, which is what led me to vegetarianism at seventeen; my relatives were dropping like flies while I was growing up.

I ran into Dr. John McDougall (www.drmcdougall.com) at an event and asked him why my cholesterol had gone as high as 212 and if it was just my bad genes. After all, I was on a basically low-fat, vegan diet. And he said, "Fructose." I said, "Well, my blood sugar is fine; it's just my cholesterol . . ." And Dr. McDougall said, "Fructose." He's a very efficient guy—he gave me a one-word diagnosis. It was like the "plastics" scene from *The Graduate*. I don't know if there's another doctor in America who would have instructed me that my problem was fructose, and certainly there isn't another who could have helped me in just one second. Other doctors would have put me on drugs and run countless tests on me and increased my stress level. He met me at a party and said "fructose." Arguably, I owe him my life.

I went home and Googled "fructose and cholesterol" and discovered that indeed there was a theory that there was a direct relationship.[5] So I experimented. For the next several weeks, instead of having for breakfast commercial, organic fruit-flavored soy yogurt, which comes sweetened with cane sugar, into which I had typically added fruits and raisins, I had oatmeal with oat bran, cut out the cookies and the soy ice cream, and cut out dried fruit. I made *absolutely no other changes.* Seven weeks later my cholesterol was 146 and my triglycerides dropped from 203 to 81. But the reason I mention this is that after I went cold turkey on the sweets for a couple months, now if I try to eat one of those cookies that I used to eat, it tastes too sweet to me. It doesn't taste good.

PP: Well, you bring up a really good point, which is the neuro-adaptation of the taste buds over time. I'm the same way. I went to a wedding of a very good friend of mine. We made the cake—Wellness Forum Foods made the cake, so it was a vegan cake. I had a tiny bit of the frosting, and it was unpleasantly sweet. I ate a couple of bites of the cake without the frosting and didn't finish it. It wasn't because we don't make good cakes. I mean, everybody else was licking the plate and looking around for more, so I know the cake was really good.

I really am a lot happier with fruit, even though I find I still have a bit of a sweet tooth. The evenings in particular are when I feel like I want something, but I'm just as happy with a nice crisp apple or a bowl of pineapple or strawberries. A bowl of strawberries makes me perfectly happy; I really don't miss the other stuff. And speaking of Dr. McDougall, he often says in his lectures that humans do have a sweet tooth and nature builds in a great way to satisfy it; it's called fruit. Go have some and you will find that you don't have to have all this other garbage.

GM: Now, in my case, Pam, I more or less cut sweets cold turkey. When people have very unhealthy diets, do you find that it's more effective for them to make major dietary changes right away, just stop what they were doing before and do something radically different, or is it more effective for people to change gradually? Or does that depend on the individual?

PP: I think the best thing to do is make a great big leap into the land of what we call dietary excellence. There are a couple of reasons for it. The first one is that, if you want to get people to stick with this—and that's my goal; I want people to do it and keep with it for the rest of their lives—they've got to see results. You know, people read *Prevention* magazine and go to their cardiologist, who will tell them to eat more fish and eat less chicken. So they work at this, making small changes to include a little more of this food, a little less of that food. They try hard, but at the end of the day, they're in worse shape from a weight and health perspective than they were before they started. That's not much motivation to keep paying attention to diet.

GM: Which could be why the medical establishment often downplays the role of diet.

PP: Yes, because they don't see results from the minimal, half-assed dietary changes they typically recommend. So I found that when we make great big changes, we see great big results, and the motivation lasts. You give somebody some phenomenal results and you don't see them going back. They'll experiment with some junk food—I call it going off the reservation—and then they'll find out how poorly they feel eating some of this stuff. They're pretty compliant after that. If we want people to be compliant, we've got to show them great results. That only happens when they do the whole diet.

I was explaining this to somebody recently. Everywhere I go, food becomes the subject of conversation. I was at my friend's wedding, sitting at this table full of people—none of whom eat like I do—and they were all curious about the way that I eat. They were saying things like, "I cut out this and that and I haven't lost a pound." "My cholesterol is still high." "I still have to take blood pressure medication." And so on. I explained to them that diet is like a combination lock. If you have to dial four numbers to open a combination lock and you dial three correctly, you don't get 75 percent of the results. You get nothing until you get that fourth number right. We have a society filled with people who are doing 75 percent of what they need to do or 50 percent of what they need to do. They don't get 50 percent or 75 percent of the results; nothing happens until they get the whole thing right.

GM: As with me. I was doing most everything right, but I was taking in too much sugar.

PP: That's why we teach dietary pattern. We really work to make people leave their old life behind and embrace dietary excellence. If we produce the changes for them that they're looking for, they'll stick with it. There's another issue, too, and it goes back to these bad foods calling their names from the kitchen. As long as the stuff is around, as long as they're teasing themselves with it every day, they're going to revert to their old ways. It's just going to go on forever. So we tell them, "Look, if you're going do this, then let's do it. Get rid of the stuff."

GM: What would you say are the most outrageous and self-destructive nutritional habits of Americans?

14

PP: Milk drinking would be right up there. All cow's milk products: cheese, butter, yogurt, cottage cheese, skim milk, all that stuff.

Call me crazy, but I find the idea of consuming another mammal's secretions kind of gross. Here's how I recommend thinking about it: all cow's milk has estrogen metabolites because it comes from lactating cows.[6] So the next time you're getting ready to put a slice of cheese on a sandwich, just think, "I'm really looking forward to a big slice of estrogen between my slices of bread." Next time you're getting ready to put skim milk on your cereal, say, "I'd really love to have estrogen with my Cheerios this morning." Doesn't that sound delightful?

GM: So how does the estrogen in cow's milk affect women who consume dairy products?

PP: Most breast cancers are estrogen receptor positive, so elevated blood levels of estrogen increase the risk of breast cancer. There's also another issue. Cow's milk is designed to help a calf grow to several hundred pounds within a short period of time, so cow's milk increases production of a hormone called insulin-like growth factor, or IGF-1, which helps to fuel this growth.[7] But dairy products also increase IGF-1 levels in humans; the dairy industry's own studies show this.[8] The problem is that IGF-1 is a powerful cancer promoter in humans; there are clear links between IGF-1 levels and breast, lung, colon, and prostate cancers. In fact, the link between low-fat cow's milk and prostate cancer is stronger than the link between smoking and lung cancer.[9]

Estrogen levels in milk increase during the cow's pregnancy. Farmers aren't supposed to milk their cows during the last two months of pregnancy, when estrogen levels are highest, but milk products still contain lots of estrogen. So that's why I'd say that consuming dairy is right up there as one of the most pernicious and dangerous dietary practices.

GM: What are some of the other worst practices?

15

PP: Drinking calories is another terrible dietary practice. I spoke at a large local school about improving foods in the school system. They've already made one very important advance: the kids can buy only water to drink. Water is the only drink available to them other than the milk that's unfortunately served with the lunch. The milk, of course, is a disaster, but at least if the kids want to buy something in the vending machines, it's water or nothing. And the reason that's important is that one thing all nutritionists pretty much agree upon is that liquid calories don't reduce the calories consumed in food. There are so many people consuming soft drinks, sports drinks, flavored milk, and juices—we're talking between 500 and 700 calories a day that don't reduce by a single calorie what they're consuming in solid foods. That's certainly one reason why people develop weight problems; drinking calories is a major contributor to obesity.

The other major dietary nightmares in the United States are too much protein, too much fat, and too little fiber, with animal foods a leading cause of all three problems. In the fat category, oil is a close second with the havoc it causes on the body.

I'll add one more thing that's become an issue in recent years: taking supplements instead of eating well. The justification for that approach is, "I know I don't eat well, but I'll just take some pills. That'll make up for my dietary indiscretions." Unfortunately, the pills people take depend on which practitioners they go to and which magazines they read; they're all fairly useless most of the time, but some of them can be dangerous.

I'd say that not understanding the importance of dietary pattern is the overarching issue. People think that they're going to improve their diets by eating soy twice a week. Or they read an article saying blueberries can reduce the risk of cancer, so they eat blueberries every day for six months. They end up gaining four pounds, and their health deteriorates because it turns out that neither blueberries nor any other single food can fix what's wrong with them. It's only by changing the fundamental dietary pattern that they can fix what's wrong. Those are some of the ways in which Americans have gone astray, why they're so confused and frustrated.

GM: Do you see supplements as an attempt to get by with minimal changes?

PP: Yes. It goes along with Americans' unending quest to eat a healthier version of their bad diets. "I'm eating chicken and fish instead of beef. I'm drinking skim milk instead of whole milk. I use only organic, cold-pressed olive oil." Well, it doesn't matter what kind of oil. Again, you need to understand the dietary pattern that promotes health. It's the entire diet that the average person eats, including many of my very well-educated friends who believe they're eating healthfully. It's their entire diet that's appalling from the standpoint of both macronutrients (protein, carbohydrate, and fat) and micronutrients (vitamins, minerals, and phytochemicals).

GM: I read about a study showing that 90 percent of Americans believe they eat a healthy diet.

PP: Yeah. Isn't that amazing? Then it must be just the other 10 percent responsible for the 40 percent obesity rate.

GM: Don't you hate it when a small minority ruins it for everyone else?

PP: People have the idea that they can eat whatever they want because it tastes good; they have no concept of the relationship between diet and human health. You see this in young people, too. Young people especially assume that they're invincible.

They think they can eat, drink, and be merry, with no price to pay. And then one day, there is. They go to the doctor and realize they've gained twenty or thirty or fifty pounds, and their cholesterol is out of control. There's a complete disregard, even in the medical community, for the idea that what goes into your mouth influences your health. That's the root of the problem.

GM: I've got a candidate for the worst food out there. I saw this on a Sunday morning news show. At the Iowa State Fair, the big hit this year was deep-fried butter.

PP: Deep-fried butter?

GM: On a stick. Four ounces of butter deep-fried, dipped in honey, and topped with a sugary glaze.

PP: Does it come with an angioplasty?

GM: The reporter, Jake Tapper, who's an intelligent guy, took a bite out of it on television, as if he thought it was amusing. He was showing us he was a good sport, a man of the people. I'll bet he has a great life as a major media figure in Washington, and I'm sure he'd like to attend his children's weddings one day, but there he was, eating deep-fried, sugar-glazed butter. Now, if he was doing a story on crystal meth being all the rage in Iowa, I don't think he'd sample it.

PP: That's what I'm saying. It's this eat, drink, and be merry approach to foods that are poisons that is truly deadly.

GM: I'm curious what first step you ask people to take to begin their dietary transformations. When people join The Wellness Forum and they are obese and on cholesterol medication, having a kitchen loaded with meat, cheese, soda pop, cookies, and chips, do you tell them to just go home and throw everything out?

PP: I tell them to take it to a church or food bank. There are people who are hungry and are worried not about cardiovascular disease and diabetes but about feeding their kids. So the best gift you can make is to take that food that doesn't serve you anymore and give it to people who desperately need food tonight. Then go buy the right stuff. We have to get over some of the mental images associated with this: I spent all this money on food and don't want to throw it out or give it away! Well, if you end up having a heart attack tomorrow, are you going to say, "Hey, I'm so glad I ate that bacon and got my money's worth. Sure, I had a heart attack, but I didn't waste a nickel!" Nobody ever sits in my office as a result of making bad choices and ending up in a bad health situation and says, "Yeah, I know I've got this breast cancer, lupus, or diabetes now, but it was so worth it because all that animal food and processed food was delicious." Get the stuff out of your house. Leave it behind. Leave your old life behind and join me. Let me take your hand and take a giant leap over to where the healthy people live.

If I could find a way to make people understand this quickly and easily, I know I'd be a billionaire. If I could develop a pill where people could live inside my body for just twenty-four hours and then go back to their own, we'd have no trouble convincing people to eat like this because they would feel how great it is to feel alive and energetic and to be able to run around eighteen hours a day. I want them to experience that. That's the only way we're going to get compliance. That's the only way people are going to get with the program.

THE PROGRAM

GM: Let's talk about the optimal diet. There's a theory out there that we're all different and we should choose our diet according to our blood type or our genetic makeup or our personality type or our astrological sign, and that the optimal diet is one thing for one person and a vastly different thing for another person. Is there any truth to the idea that different people need wildly different diets, or are we mostly alike in what we ought to be eating?

PP: We're shockingly alike. The only thing that differentiates us significantly is food allergies. My attorney, who died a couple years ago at sixty-one, was in his fifties when I met him. He had been allergic to cherries, peaches, and apricots since he was five. Well, he could eat a plant-based diet, but since cherries, peaches, and apricots sent him into anaphylactic shock, we kept him away from those foods. That would be an example of a genetic situation; stay away from three specific foods.

GM: Wait a minute. He ate a plant-based diet, but died at sixty-one?

PP: Well, he cheated a lot. He died of noncompliance. He would say he was on a plant-based diet, but he never gave up cheeses and salmon, and he ate olive oil and sweets. One day it caught up with him and he had a massive heart attack. He was a successful man and he liked to live large; as a consequence, he died in an instant. It was a tragic example of how you have to get the whole diet right, not just get half of the equation right.

But with reference to this idea that people are different and therefore some people should eat different types of diets because of their ethnicity or their blood type, there's no solid evidence. I come to all my conclusions based on medical evidence. If you wonder whether there's anything to the blood-type diet, do PubMed searches. Anybody can do it. You'll find absolutely no published evidence indicating that blood type makes a difference in long-term health outcomes. I get very frustrated because the promoters of these blood type diets and metabolic diets and caveman diets have made millions and millions of dollars promoting these programs to patients and the general public. And they spend none of that money on proving their hypotheses. I love the way Dr. T. Colin Campbell, the author of *The China Study*, put it when he was going head-to-head on the Internet with someone who was criticizing him: "Put your theory to the test because what you're essentially saying by refusing to do so is that research is a luxury to be enjoyed by some but not required by all." And that's a rather insulting attitude to those of us who are serious because I, for one, rigorously adhere to what the science says about all aspects of nutrition. There simply isn't a shred of evidence that the caveman diet or these other fad diets help achieve or maintain optimal health in populations today. These people are writing storybooks. They may be very interesting, but they're not to be confused with science. They cite a lot of studies, but a close look shows that they misinterpret them to promote their diet, and they never conduct a single study of their own to prove their case.

Let me give you an example of how storytelling can confuse the issue. When I conduct lectures, invariably I'll have somebody raise his hand and say, "My uncle ate bacon, eggs, and cheese three times a day and he lived to be ninety-four and died in his sleep. How do you explain that?" And I will say, "I believe you. I believe that happened. But if you delve into the published scientific information that we have, it clearly shows that is not the likely outcome for other people who engage in that behavior." So that's a story. It's probably a true story. It has nothing to do with the advice that we should give to the general population.

GM: You've got to love the premise of the caveman diet books, that we should, for some reason, eat the diet of our primitive ancestors. Maybe to prove that civilization has not come that far. I actually have a theory that the first vegan was a caveman who discovered that it's easier to sneak up on a plant.

Anyway, since we're shockingly alike as humans, what should our diet be? Let's begin with fat. What percentage of calories from fat should we have in our diet? There are those who recommend a plant-based diet and emphasize that it should be low-fat, roughly 10 percent of calories as fat. And there are others, even some who recommend the vegan diet, who say no, we need a healthy amount of nuts and seeds and avocados, a higher percentage of fat. And then, of course, there are the diet book hucksters, like Dr. Barry Sears and the late Dr. Robert Atkins, who promote a diet that's 30 percent fat or more.

PP: Let's disregard the hucksters because they're not worth our time. But between the serious scientists advocating a low-fat, plant-based diet and the serious scientists advocating a plant-based diet that's somewhat higher in fat, I think the answer is in the middle. I don't like to restrict people more than is necessary; my general recommendation to people is an upper limit of 15 percent, which is still pretty low. It's very achievable if we get oils out of the diet and use nuts and seeds and olives and avocados as parts of dishes that we eat, but don't go out of our way to eat a bunch of fatty plant foods all the time. Now, for somebody who has coronary artery disease, or who needs to lose a hundred pounds, we want to get him down to the 9 to 11 percent range in terms of fat, which means he's not going to be consuming avocados and nuts and olives. I recommend an upper limit of 15 percent and a lower limit of 9 to 11 percent for people who have certain kinds of diseases.

GM: Allow me to cite a mainstream nutritionist: Walter Willett of the Harvard School of Public Health. He argues that low-fat diets show no improvement in health outcomes compared with higher-fat diets; the important thing is to have good fats—polyunsaturated and monounsaturated fat. He cites a *Journal of the American Medical Association* study published in 2006,[1] an eight-year study of more than 49,000 women that he says demonstrated no improvement in outcomes from a low-fat diet.

PP: Willett is not the only person who finds that a low-fat diet does not provide benefit. The problem is his definition of a low-fat diet, and definitions are something that plague nutritional research. In Willett's Nurse's Study, for example (I think the government has invested roughly a hundred million dollars in this whole project), the lowest amount of fat these women ever consumed was in the vicinity of 29 or 30 percent! I don't think any of us who advocate a plant-based diet has ever told anybody that a diet that contains 30 percent of calories as fat is protective against anything. The other thing I'll point out about Willett's research and the Nurse's Study is that one of the ways in which people accomplish a "low-fat" diet is often to eat fat-free dairy products. The detrimental effect of the concentrated protein in those dairy products often overcomes the benefit of any fat reduction, even if it were to reach the target level.

GM: Okay, so let's say I'm convinced that I should aim for roughly 10 to 15 percent of my calories as fat. How do I execute that? I couldn't tell you with any accuracy the percentage of calories I ingest is fat. Are you recommending that people somehow count their calories and calculate the percentage derived from fat?

PP: I tell people, if you're eating according to our pyramid, you'll be just fine. I can't teach people to be either calorie counters or nutrient counters because it can't be done. And I use myself as an example. Today for lunch I had a salad with one of Wellness Forum Chef Del Sroufe's fat-free dressings and a rice and vegetable casserole. So I had a nice big portion of this casserole and a big plate of salad with dressing. In order for me to tell you how many calories I ate, I'd have to come back here to my office with a database and feed in fairly accurate information about how many pieces of broccoli I ate, how much rice was on the plate, and how much dressing I put on the salad. Of course I would have no clue. So if somebody like me, with my background in nutrition and my resources, can't figure out what I had for lunch from a calorie and nutrient standpoint, how do we take a busy CPA who's preparing somebody's tax return and teach her to do it on a lunch break? It's obviously not doable.

What you have to do is teach the right dietary pattern. Just stay attuned to the principles of the diet. The only way you're going to mess it up is if you start treating yourself all the time, or the oils start creeping into the diet and you start eating those items at the top of the pyramid with a great deal of liberalism. But if you stick with the basic food groups that we're talking about, you'll get full, you won't develop a weight problem, and you'll lose weight if you need to. You just can't overeat. I couldn't have possibly eaten another plate of food today; it would have been too much bulk.

THE WELLNESS FORUM'S
Eating Plan

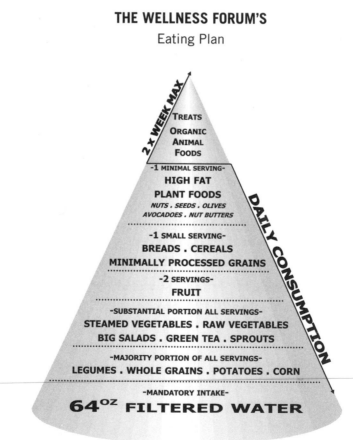

2 X WEEK MAX

TREATS
ORGANIC
ANIMAL
FOODS

-1 MINIMAL SERVING-
HIGH FAT
PLANT FOODS
NUTS . SEEDS . OLIVES
AVOCADOES . NUT BUTTERS

-1 SMALL SERVING-
BREADS . CEREALS
MINIMALLY PROCESSED GRAINS

-2 SERVINGS-
FRUIT

-SUBSTANTIAL PORTION ALL SERVINGS-
STEAMED VEGETABLES . RAW VEGETABLES
BIG SALADS . GREEN TEA . SPROUTS

-MAJORITY PORTION OF ALL SERVINGS-
LEGUMES . WHOLE GRAINS . POTATOES . CORN

-MANDATORY INTAKE-
64^{OZ} FILTERED WATER

DAILY CONSUMPTION

GM: We've discussed fat. How about protein? I find that when people talk about nutrition, their concerns tend to be their weight and their protein intake. Do you find that's what people are most concerned about?

PP: Those are two major anxieties, but people have lots of misdirected concerns. I have people coming into my office with serious health and weight problems, and they're worried about the plastic in water bottles and about all kinds of things that may be concerning but they're hardly the main issue. Americans are very distracted by information that isn't pertinent at the expense of getting to the information that is pertinent.

People are concerned about their weight, but not enough of them, in my opinion. There's an interesting phenomenon going on in our country and it's the way that we've simply accepted our increasing weight. When I was in high school, there were more than seven hundred kids in our graduating class and only a handful of them were overweight. Now most of the students in graduating classes are overweight. People who are overweight look around and everyone looks like them; they don't feel particularly bad about it or feel compelled to do something about it right away. And that's an insidious trend because being overweight puts you at additional risk for every disease you don't want to get and for dying from those diseases.

Regarding protein: it's all but impossible to design a diet that has enough calories every day that doesn't contain enough protein because protein needs are so low. Excretion studies have shown that protein needs for normal adults may be as low as 2.5 percent of calories.[2] Human breast milk, which fuels most rapid growth of humans during our entire time on the planet, contains only 6 percent protein.[3] So there's not much chance of protein deficiency in any diet of caloric sufficiency. I've told people, just go to the USDA food database and start entering any combination of foods that add up to 1,500 or 2,000 calories a day; you're going to see that it's impossible to become protein deficient eating any combination of food. Our problem, by contrast, is that we eat way too much protein.

GM: What's the risk there?

PP: We now know that animal protein consumed in excess of what humans need becomes a powerful cancer promoter, based on Dr. Campbell's studies as reported in *The China Study*.[4] Even if you consumed a really high-protein, plant-based diet, the fact remains that the body's need for protein is actually very low. So if you consume too much protein, even plant protein, you simply have to get rid of the excess; we can't store much protein. What the body will do is convert some of the surplus protein to carbohydrate because that's readily usable for energy. In the process of doing this, the body has to get rid of nitrogen from the amino acid chains, as carbohydrate does not include nitrogen.[5] As the body releases nitrogen from the amino acid chains, the nitrogen throws off a lot of toxic by-products like urea and ammonia, which are detoxified by the kidneys and liver, causing a lot of stress on those organs.

GM: So we basically have this word—protein—that enjoys a great reputation. We have whole industries that are set up to provide us with an abundance of protein, whether it's in the form of a snack bar or a highly concentrated protein supplement. And you're saying that it's really just a myth that all this protein is good for you? That if protein had the lousy public relations guy that starch has, we might not have all these protein bars in health food stores?

PP: Yes, and we would be healthier. The myth goes back, as I learned from Dr. Campbell, to protein's origin as one of the first nutrients discovered. A lot of benefit was attributed to it because if you withheld protein from lab animals, they died. It was around 1839 when protein was discovered, and researchers at the time attributed all this magical quality to it. *My gosh, without it people will die!* And that's true—it's a necessary nutrient—but they exaggerated the benefit, especially by assuming that since a little is indispensable, a lot must be salutary. The belief never got corrected, even when evidence began to show that their inferences were wrong. Russell Chittenden did some experiments back in the early 1900s on students eating a low-protein diet and found that they thrived; even the athletes performed better on it.[6] But once an idea takes hold and becomes part of the conventional wisdom in the health field, it is very hard to undo. It's very frustrating. People in the health field are not easily persuaded by facts.

GM: I have a friend who told me that he eats meat for protein to build muscle. I pointed out that elephants manage to grow pretty strong on a diet of plants. This gave him pause. He pondered for a long while and then said, "Yeah, but I don't want to get fat."

Muscle builders will generally eat a high-protein diet. They'll have egg whites and fortified protein foods because they believe it helps them bulk up. Are they right about that, that it helps them develop muscle?

PP: Well, if protein built muscle, if you could build muscle in the kitchen, we'd live in a land full of Arnold Schwarzeneggers. The issue with bodybuilders is something I call error of attribution. In other words, bodybuilders need more food and more calories, but it doesn't necessarily mean that they need more protein. However, when they start doing aggressive bodybuilding and athletic activities, their coaches and advisors tell them to increase their protein intake; they do and they feel better as a result. But what they're really doing is adding the extra calories that they need to their diets; they would feel equally well if they ate a diet like the one that you and I eat.

GM: So their muscles could get just as big on our diet?

PP: Yes, because the way muscles get big is resistance training, which is somewhat limited to gender and genetic predisposition. There is nothing that most men can do to look like an NFL linebacker. They'll just never have that body type, no matter how much they exercise, no matter how much they eat. We do have genetic limitations, but it is possible for somebody with the right genes to become just as big or strong by eating a plant-centered diet. (Interested parties can check out www.veganbodybuilding.com.)

Athletes may be the key to turning popular opinion around because what they do is high profile and they're always looking for an edge. There are some pretty high-profile athletes who have converted to a plant-based diet and their performances improved. The triathlete Dave Scott was vegan when he won six Ironman Triathlons in the 1980s. Carl Lewis was vegan when he was setting track records, and he attributes his success to the vegan diet. And then there's Tony Gonzalez, one of the older players in the NFL, who adopted a plant-based diet.

GM: There are more and more vegan athletes all the time. NFL running backs Arian Foster and Montell Owens, boxer Timothy Bradley, former NBA basketball players John Salley and Salim Stoudamire, tennis champion Venus Williams, ultimate fighters Mac Danzig and Jake Shields, and "the world's toughest woman," Juliana Sproles, winner of the "Tough Mudder" competition.

PP: Tough Mudder bills itself as the toughest obstacle course on the planet, and it's now clear, for any who may have had doubts, that you can win it without ingesting any animal protein.

GM: Okay, so an increase in animal protein doesn't result in an increase in the size of your muscles or in improved athletic performance. What are the differences between animal protein and plant protein?

PP: Well, *The China Study* shows that the cancer-promoting effect was limited to animal protein. We didn't see this effect when it came to plant protein, but that doesn't mean that high amounts of plant protein don't become problematic. That's why people need to consume a high-carbohydrate, low-protein, low-fat diet.

GM: So we have an upper limit of 15 percent of calories from fat, and an upper limit of 10 percent from protein. By my math, I'd say we're talking a lower limit of 75 percent from carbohydrate?

PP: Yes, from whole, unprocessed foods. Legumes, vegetables (including the starchy vegetables), fruit, and whole grains. Fiber-rich foods are the basis of the diet. Not the carbohydrates found in processed foods, fruit juices, and sugar. The label "carb" gets applied in common usage to both unhealthy processed foods and healthy whole grain foods and vegetables; that's why it's important to focus on eating whole plant foods and forget about the useless label "carbs."

GM: Let's get more specific about your dietary plan. What do you advise that people eat for their three meals a day?

PP: Well, first of all, I don't advise eating just three meals a day. We have them eat four or five or even six meals a day. I want them to do that for a couple of reasons. The first is that I don't want people getting ravenous because it leads to overeating. If you eat breakfast at 6:30 in the morning and don't eat lunch until 12:30, you're likely to be so ravenous by the time you sit down for lunch that you're going to overeat. While it's not that you want to eat when you're not hungry, you want to eat when you're beginning to get mildly hungry; for most people, that's every three or four hours or so. The second thing is that when your blood sugar levels get low enough, if you really wait until you're out of fuel, you won't feel or think well. I like to get up in the morning and operate with high-speed cognitive ability and energy all day long; that's really hard to do when your system's completely empty. So we like four, five, six meals a day, with smaller amounts of food at each meal than one would consume on a three-meal-per-day plan.

And we like to offer people specific suggestions for what to eat for breakfast. Oatmeal is always good and it's really simple. Oatmeal and raisins, for example, and a sliced banana. Or I make a fruit smoothie in the morning that has vegetable powders, almond milk, a banana, frozen berries, some flaxseeds, food-grade green tea, and brewer's yeast. You might wonder what's up with brewer's yeast and vegetable powders. I'm all about maximizing my intake of superfoods—chopping up kale and adding it to soup, using romaine lettuce to make wraps instead of tortillas, for example. So I had Wellness Forum Foods develop a smoothie mix with simple ingredients—dehydrated vegetable powders in the morning is a good thing—brewer's yeast because it is such a concentrated source of several vitamins and minerals; food-grade green tea, which is a powerful source of antioxidants; and flax seeds. Mix in a blender with almond milk, a banana, and some frozen fruit, and you have a nice twenty-ounce drink with fourteen grams of fiber. It tastes kind of like a milkshake with frozen fruit in it. I look forward to it every morning.

I know people who like rice and vegetables for breakfast, so I tell them to go for it. You don't have to wait until noon or six o'clock to have rice and vegetables. If you want a baked potato for breakfast, that's fine. We have some strange biases in this country about which foods can be eaten at which times of the day. On a typical day for me, I start with my smoothie and then I'll have some cereal midmorning. Today I had broccoli casserole and salad for lunch. If I get hungry midafternoon, I'll have some leftover broccoli casserole. For dinner, I'll have a great big salad and baked potatoes or rice and vegetables. My sweet tooth sets in during the evening, so I'm most likely to eat fruit for a snack.

That's the basic plan. It doesn't have to be fancy. I still love to go out once in a while and eat elegant food, but once your taste buds get down-regulated, you find that you're perfectly satisfied with simple fare. It's not that you don't focus on flavor—the food I eat is really delicious—but I'm happy with baked sweet potatoes and a salad. Steamed vegetables and rice and a salad. Baked potatoes and black bean soup. A lot of simple fare that's really, really good.

GM: Let's list the grains that could be the basis of a diet.

PP: Rice, quinoa, wheat, corn, barley, buckwheat, any of them.

GM: Now, wheat is something people generally eat in the form of bread, pasta, and couscous—

PP: Right, but wheat berries are also swell. I wish I ate more of them, actually, because they're really good. They're very filling and people generally like them; they're kind of chewy and have a great texture.

GM: You make it like you make rice. You just boil wheat berries?

PP: Yes, and that's an important point. People generally know what to do with rice, but they're less familiar with other grains. People say, "I know how to cook rice, but what do I do with barley or quinoa?" And the answer is, substitute it. You know how to make rice and vegetables, rice and beans, you know how to put a cup of rice in soup—do the same thing with barley, quinoa, buckwheat, wheat berries, any grain. Boil it just as you would boil rice and use it the same way in the meal. That gets people experimenting with different grains. And it's the simple substitution for rice that gets them to step outside their usual eating pattern a little bit. Later they take it a step further; there's an abundance of cooking classes and healthy-eating cookbooks using plant-based food. You just have to get to the place where you understand what it is you want to learn how to do. It isn't eating chicken and fish instead of beef; it's eating plants instead of animals. And once you get that distinction in your mind and understand that by "plants" we don't mean tofu hot dogs and fruit juice–sweetened cookies, you're on your way. We're talking about whole, unprocessed plant foods. It's then easy to source out information with that distinction made.

GM: Speaking of tofu, for people who are used to having chicken or fish or meat—high-protein deceased animals—as a centerpiece of their meals, how do you feel about replacing animal protein with tofu, tempeh, seitan, or some other high-protein plant food?

PP: They're fine. Over time we want to be getting closer to the beans, rice, corn, potatoes, steamed vegetables, raw vegetables, and fruit diet, rather than so much high-protein meat substitutes. It's also important to differentiate between minimally processed meat substitutes, like tofu and tempeh, versus the tofu hot dogs, fake pepperoni, and other highly processed meat substitutes that are really just vegan-friendly junk food. These junk foods are okay while you're first transitioning to a plant-based diet, or when you're going to a holiday picnic, but they should not be part of the daily fare.

34

GM: Is giving up the traditional meat, chicken, or fish the hardest part for folks?

PP: Well, sometimes they give it up for something even more deadly. At the wedding I talked about earlier, while I was eating a plate of broccoli, everybody else ate veggie lasagna. Now, veggie lasagna, you think, "Hey, that sounds pretty healthy, right? That's got to be better for you than meat." This veggie lasagna had four kinds of cheese in it and was topped with a cream sauce. And really there isn't any red meat they could've served at this place that would be more deadly than the veggie lasagna that they served as the centerpiece of the meal.

GM: Four kinds of cheese and cream? That's not really a whole lot better than deep-fried butter on a stick.

PP: Exactly. At best we're talking only a difference of degree between what health-conscious, sophisticated people at an urban wedding are eating and the crap that we think only unsophisticated rubes would eat. So the centerpiece of the meal can be something that appears to be healthy and often isn't. I've been at people's houses when they've said, "Oh, we know you're a vegetarian, so we made a vegetarian meal for you." And they serve pasta and vegetables. I figure, okay, that's not bad, how can you mess that up, right? Well, if I take pasta and vegetables and douse it in olive oil, I've just consumed enough fat for the week in one meal. So even people trying to accommodate me on a vegan plan mess it up, despite the best of intentions.

GM: Would you say that, in addition to a surfeit of unhealthy ingredients, like dairy products and meats and oil and sugar, Americans suffer from a lack of nutrients that they need?

PP: Yes, and that happens in a couple of different ways, actually. For example, people take in gargantuan amounts of salt on the standard American diet and virtually no potassium. And it's not just the excess salt that's the problem; the lack of potassium is a problem, too. So they adapt a plant-based diet, potassium levels go up, salt consumption goes down, and the body is much healthier. People overconsume some nutrients and underconsume others. A lot of people in this country are overfed, but are still malnourished. Also, people who eat the standard American diet generally have pretty messed-up gastrointestinal tracts due to constipation and inflammation. That makes it difficult for them to absorb the nutrients that they're taking in. So the nutrient deficiencies happen two ways: what they're putting (or not putting, actually) in their mouths and how much of it actually gets into the system.

GM: Let's talk about inflammation. Inflammation can be systemic, is that right? If your body gets inflamed, it's throughout the tissues of the body?

PP: Yes. You could have localized inflammation. You have surgery and the site of the incision becomes inflamed; there are some things you can do about that, and we all understand that. Inflammation can also be generalized, which we can measure with something called a CRP test, for C-reactive protein. It doesn't tell you where the inflammation is, but the most likely place is the lining of the blood vessels, the endothelial cells that produce nitric oxide and keep the blood vessels open. That's usually where the inflammation resides, which is why CRP is considered a pretty good marker for a risk of coronary artery disease.

GM: What's causing this inflammation?

PP: Animal foods contain something called arachidonic acid. In small amounts, it's really not so bad for you. However when you consume a lot of it, it's a precursor to something called series-2 prostaglandins, which are inflammatory. Again, it's good to produce some series-2 prostaglandins; too much, though, and you get some inflammation. So that's one way some inflammation happens.

Another cause of inflammation is obesity itself. We used to think that adipose cells and tissues were just sort of benign and didn't do much; now we know that these cells are busy all day long pumping out substances like hormones and inflammatory cytokines. So the fat cells of overweight people are pumping out inflammatory chemicals all day long, leading to generalized inflammation. That's why it's so important to address the weight issue. Even a person eating a plant-based or vegan diet can be maintaining extra weight and is therefore still at high risk for lots of health issues.

GM: How does CRP rank as a marker of heart disease compared with cholesterol and homocysteine?

PP: They're all good markers and they all should be low numbers. Cholesterol should be under 150 mg/dl, CRP should be 1.5 mg/L or lower, and homocysteine under 6 micro mol/L. So you want low numbers all the way around. But here's the big problem: we've gotten to the place now where we focus on those numbers and don't necessarily care how we get there. People go to the doctor and they're diagnosed with high biomarkers. The doctor puts them on drugs to bring those numbers down without actually changing the health status of the individual. And what's the result? A new phenomenon in this country, as Dr. McDougall points out: people dying of sudden heart attacks with great blood work.

GM: The classic good news, bad news kind of thing.

PP: It's sad but true. Instead of curing the individual, we're curing his biomarkers. Here's an example to illustrate how terrible our system is. Tim Russert, NBC News' political guru, died a few years ago. He had a great job, great insurance, and money. He went to the best doctors and had all the right tests done. He was diagnosed early, which is supposed to be a good thing, right? He was treated for all his problems: he took a drug for blood pressure, statin drugs, a drug to treat his pre-diabetic condition, and a daily aspirin. And he still died at fifty-eight of a heart attack because none of those drugs addressed what was wrong with him: the amount of unstable plaques throughout his arteries from the animal food and fat that he was eating. He trusted his doctors and they offered what Western medicine traditionally offers, which did him no good at all.

On the other hand, you get the critics of the Western pharmaceutical approach, the advocates of a more holistic approach to pharmacology, who say that Russert shouldn't have been taking those drugs. Instead, they say he should have been taking high-dose cinnamon for his diabetes, hawthorn berry for his blood pressure, and high-dose niacin or red rice yeast extract for his cholesterol. And you know what? He'd still be a dead guy with great blood work because none of those things address what killed him. So, we've gotten very carried away with biomarkers. While we need to look at them, we also need to recognize that all methods to bring them down aren't equal. The only thing that brings those numbers down in a way that matters is diet. The other things change your blood work, but don't change your health outcome.

GM: I remember when Tim Russert died; all his colleagues talked about what a great guy he was and how they loved going to the ball game with him and having hot dogs together. Of course, they didn't seem aware of the irony that it was those very hot dogs that helped cause his death.

PP: Right, and unfortunately, he just dropped dead. Other people survive a heart attack and end up going to the average dietician or cardiologist, who tell them to eat fish and lean meats and poultry. Their cholesterol keeps going up, so the doctors say, "Well, you know, it's a genetic issue." The doctors put them on a pharmaceutical drug because that's really all they know to do.

If people really understood, in clear terms, what food did to them, they'd have a whole different attitude about it. I know when people come to my lectures, they leave with a whole different attitude. They don't all change overnight, but they leave with a different attitude about the whole thing.

GM: What's their attitude about giving up the animal foods that they grew up eating and have been encouraged to eat all their lives?

PP: Well, first of all, at The Wellness Forum, we don't ask people to give up animal foods entirely. The Wellness Forum is not an explicitly or exclusively vegan program.

GM: Okay. Why not?

PP: Because I've yet to see the evidence that people who eat a low-fat, starch-centered, plant-based diet, while including up to three servings a week of animal foods, have worse health outcomes than people on a similar, but purely vegan, diet. There just is no such evidence. I believe, and my experience with The Wellness Forum confirms my belief, that we will help more people convert to a healthy diet if we espouse a more moderate message, if we don't scare people away by insisting that they abstain from animal foods entirely.

Now when I say "moderate," I'm not repeating the shibboleth that everything in moderation is okay, like cheeseburgers and ice cream sundaes; I'm saying that it's not a dealbreaker to have two or three small servings—three to five ounces—per week of wild-caught salmon or organically raised beef. There's no wiggle room on the diet; when we say two or three servings, that doesn't mean four or five or six, and dairy is absolutely out. And it's important that, if you choose to include two or three portions of animal foods per week, that they be from organically raised animals or wild-caught fish, which in almost all cases is going to mean that you're going to have to prepare these meals at home.

Let's not forget that we have this phenomenon of the un-healthy vegan. There are a lot of people who've renounced animal foods for ethical reasons. I respect their decision; that's an admirable reason to give up animal foods. I have no quarrel with their reasoning, but many of these people are no healthier than their meat-eating counterparts. They're living on veggie cheeses, fake meats, olive oil, margarine, potato chips, and French fries. You'll be much better off from a health standpoint if you eat according to The Wellness Forum program, even if you choose to include two or three portions of organically raised meat per week, than if you eat a fat-laden, nutrient-poor vegan diet.

GM: I'll accept that yours may well be the most effective approach to getting people to convert to a healthy diet; I just won't go so far as to actually endorse eating any animal foods, since I believe that the optimal intake of such foods is zero.

People make their dietary decisions based on lots of factors, including convenience, taste, and habit. And to the extent that for any or all of these reasons, people decide to continue to consume some animal products in accordance with The Wellness Forum guidelines, I have no issue with that. But for those who are making their dietary decisions strictly based on health concerns, here's what I would say: there is no direct scientific evidence that small amounts of flesh foods in the diet will have a detrimental effect on your health or your longevity. Indeed, some of the longest-lived populations, like the Okinawans, eat fish. But since we know that all flesh foods, including fish, have no fiber, are high in fat and cholesterol, are high in sulfuric animal protein, contain no antioxidants, and have no carbohydrate for the fueling of our cells, we might want to deduce that if you consume a little of it, to the extent that it affects your health at all, it might be in a negative way. At least, that's my reasoning.

PP: Glen, you've made a personal choice. What you're saying is, "It's better for me to have no animal foods at all." I've made the same choice. I just don't want to say that's the only choice available, or that one has to make that choice in order to achieve and maintain optimal health.

GM: Do you come across people who say, "I can try this Wellness Forum diet, but only because I can still have my chicken or fish a couple of times a week"? And then a year or two later they go vegan?

PP: Yes, lots of them. We call them the accidental vegans. We can almost tell in advance who they're going to be. It's an interesting thing; it's the people who are most likely to draw the line in the sand and say, "I don't want to be a vegan!" We tell them that we're not asking them to be vegan. And then they make that decision on their own later on and announce it proudly. I'm an accidental vegan myself, by the way.

GM: Are you?

PP: Yeah. When I first converted to this diet, I still allowed myself to have fish a couple of times a month. I did that for a while and then more or less forgot about the fish. One day I woke up and

41

said, "Huh, I don't think I've had fish for six or seven months."
And then I thought, "Well, apparently I don't miss it, so I don't
think I'm going to have it anymore."

GM: Let's stipulate that people are drawn to the vegan diet not
just for reasons of health but also out of concern for the treatment
of animals and for the environment. Half of the United States
right now is suffering a severe drought; the grazing of animals
contributes to drought by reducing vegetation, from which water
transpires.[7] Animal agriculture has been determined by a United
Nations report to be the world's leading source of greenhouse
gases,[8] and it's a leading cause of water pollution; in countless
ways, it's creating an environmental nightmare. But I think we
can also agree that the animal agriculture industry would worry
more about 30 or 40 or 50 percent of the population scaling back
to just a couple of servings of meat per week than it would worry
about 1 or 2 or 3 percent of the population going strictly vegan.

PP: If half of the country ate animal food only a couple of times
a week, and only organic animal food, the factory farms would be
gone. You'd have some humane, small operations out there, but
factory farming would not be remotely sustainable with such reduced demand. And if we could encourage millions of Americans
to eat this way, the improvement in their health will encourage
millions more, and a tipping point would be reached. And from
that pool of enlightened people, there's no telling how many accidental vegans might be created.

GM: And we do know for a fact that when people eat this way,
others are inspired to join the fold because the effects are dramatic.

PP: Absolutely. People who have gone through The Wellness Forum
program have improved the quality of their lives enormously,

extended their lives, and brought new life into the world against the odds.

GM: Against the odds?

PP: Many of the members of The Wellness Forum have been women who were unable to conceive until they got on our program. We've had about a hundred babies delivered to women who hadn't been able to conceive or who had had one or more miscarriages until they found us.

GM: That's something I didn't know. This diet can help a woman conceive?

PP: Absolutely. I say that for two reasons: a lot of anecdotal evidence that I've seen here at The Wellness Forum, and clinical studies that demonstrate that the proper diet can help a woman conceive.[9,10,11]

GM: And bring more plant eaters into the world?

PP: I certainly hope so.

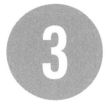

3

DISEASES AND THE FOODS THAT BRING THEM ON

....

GM: Pam, here's my nearly all-inclusive list of the various causes of diseases: diet and lifestyle, the environment, genes, stress, psychological factors, and pathogens. Let's review the many maladies plaguing our population and examine the cause for each. Let's start with heart disease.

PP: Definitely diet and lifestyle.

GM: Does genetics play any role?

PP: With very few people. I can say the same with regard to any condition that we would label chronic and degenerative. You have genetic predisposition, but those genes are switched on by diet and lifestyle choices. You're going to have, in any practice setting, 2 to 3 percent of the population whose cholesterol levels, no matter how much they clean up their diet and lifestyle, won't get down to ideal levels. Or perhaps they're salt-sensitive and an adjustment in salt intake is needed to get their blood pressure down, and sometimes even that doesn't work. We see a very tiny percentage of people who honestly have been dealt a bad hand. But the good news is that you can say to the new person coming in that the chances are outrageously high that your body is going to respond positively to this diet and lifestyle that we're going to show you and that it's well worth doing.

GM: I'm someone with heart disease and hypercholesterolemia rampant in my family, and yet I lowered my cholesterol levels when I finally got the diet exactly right.

PP: Yeah, most people have had it drilled into them that it's familial; I tell them that there's no question that you have genetic predisposition. As I think I've mentioned to you, women in my family have rheumatoid arthritis and they're fat. I'm positive that it would not take me, at my age, but a year or two to eat my way into rheumatoid arthritis and obesity, if I choose to do so. But I'm not going to switch on those bad genes with my diet.

GM: How about strokes?

PP: Definitely diet and lifestyle. There are times when there is a structural abnormality that will cause somebody to develop a blood clot. That's fairly rare; again, it's diet and lifestyle that's going to cause your risk of stroke to go up. Stroke is an outcome of atherosclerosis, just like heart disease.

GM: High blood pressure?

PP: Diet and lifestyle most of the time. The causes are similar to heart disease and stroke.

GM: Cancer?

PP: Diet and lifestyle, above all. Two lifestyle factors are significant: obviously, cigarettes profoundly increase the risk of many cancers, not just lung cancer, and alcohol increases the risk of many cancers, not just liver cancer. There's a role that stress plays, but it may not be what people think. I don't think stress causes cancer, just as I don't think it causes heart disease. I think that stress often causes people to become even less diligent about taking care of themselves; that's its role in disease-promotion. As your stress levels increase, you may exercise less, eat more junk food, or turn to alcohol, and that's how you end up with cancer.

GM: What about the environmental factor for cancer?

PP: The environment is often responsible for cancer initiation, but not usually promotion; it's diet that promotes the cancer. There *are* some types of cancer, however, that are purely environmental. For example, I had a good friend die of lung cancer who never smoked. However, he owned a plastics factory. He used to spend a lot of time on the factory floor, of course, and this was at a time when environmental regulations were a lot more lax. That's probably what caused his lung cancer. That would be a case of an environmental cause, but it's an atypical case. And you also have to consider the degree of exposure. My friend's exposure was massive and daily, as opposed to our exposure to chemical carcinogens and air pollution, which is not as massive as people might believe. I think that that's a minor factor for most people.

There is an area where environment and diet overlap concerning carcinogens—pesticides and toxins in our food. The most important thing to know about toxins is that they are concentrated in the fatty tissues of animals and become more concentrated as you move up the food chain. Fish have levels of heavy metals, pesticides, and other toxins that are often off the charts. As a general rule, you'll find far less pesticide exposure in plant foods and you can wash some of it off, or avoid it altogether if you eat plants grown organically. But even the Environmental Working Group, one of the most active in trying to change farming practices, states on its website that the benefits of eating fruits and vegetables far outweigh any exposure to pesticides in those foods.

GM: Type 1 and type 2 diabetes?

PP: Type 2 diabetes is definitely brought on by diet and lifestyle. For type 1 diabetes, there are a number of causes, but a major one is dairy products through the mechanism known as molecular mimicry.[1,2,3] Some other causes can be viruses and infections, and genetics is definitely a factor as well. In other words, we know that not all children who consume cow's milk develop juvenile diabetes, so there has to be some genetic predisposition that actually causes that to happen. Of course, we don't know which kids are genetically susceptible, so when we feed almost every child in the country cow's milk, some of them will get juvenile diabetes. The better option would be to never give cow's milk to infants and toddlers.

GM: So I take it you're an advocate for breast-feeding.

PP: I am. Dr. John McDougall says that if he were surgeon general, he would make formula available only by prescription. I'm not sure I'd go that far, but I do think we need to educate all moms-to-be that infants do best with breast milk, and there are many negative consequences of formula feeding, including compromised immunity and increased risk for many diseases, such as asthma[4] and Crohn's disease.[5]

GM: If somebody has the genetic predisposition to type 1 and he never consumes dairy, might the gene still express itself?

PP: It could, if exposed to the right virus or some types of infection.

GM: What do we know about the cause of Alzheimer's?

PP: Alzheimer's is a cardiovascular disease, very much related to diet and lifestyle.[6]

GM: Now that's not generally accepted wisdom, is it?

PP: No, it's not. I think the general wisdom about the etiology of most diseases comes down to genes, bad luck, and we don't know.

GM: Most mainstream doctors would concede that diet and lifestyle play a major role in heart disease, but they wouldn't say that about Alzheimer's.

PP: True. But their own medical journals, if they would take the time to read them, have shown that taking statin drugs can improve symptoms in early-stage Alzheimer's patients.[7] That tells me that there's a connection. The other thing is that the brain is the biggest user of glucose, oxygen, and water, so it only makes sense that if you narrow blood vessels to the brain, you're going to impair its supply of those essential substances.

GM: What about the fact that with Alzheimer's, there's an amyloid plaque that forms that resembles the plaque found in people who have Creutzfeldt-Jakob disease (CJD), the human form of mad cow disease?

PP: Yes, and there's a theory, which Howard Lyman has talked about, that some people being diagnosed with Alzheimer's actually have CJD.[8] Alzheimer's is rarely present in plant-eating populations; it's a disease of the Western diet. It's a vascular disease that is most prevalent in the populations, like ours, that eat the most meat.[9]

GM: What's the cause of osteoporosis?

PP: Well, first of all, osteoporosis is a mythical disease much of the time.

GM: It's mythical?

PP: To the extent that it actually exists, it's principally a diet and lifestyle disease, or it's drug-induced. For example, taking steroids can cause osteoporosis. Another thing that happens is people with celiac disease and gastrointestinal disorders often have osteoporosis because they are not absorbing nutrients from foods, including calcium and other nutrients, needed to build bones. But the vast majority of the time, the diagnosis of osteoporosis is fictitious.

GM: Well, could you explain that? We have millions of Americans believing they have osteoporosis and taking drugs for it. Have they imagined it? What's going on?

PP: No, they haven't imagined it; their doctors have helped them arrive at this conclusion. Years and years ago, osteoporosis would be diagnosed if somebody would have a fracture or broken bone for no apparent reason; maybe they wouldn't even know they had a fracture—they would just experience pain. Some type of X-ray or imaging would show that the cause of the pain was a fracture. Without the evidence of any impact or memory of falling down or anything else, they would consider a diagnosis of osteoporosis. They used to put you on this scanning device that was very expensive and very large. They would do a whole-body scan that would show porous bones in the skeleton and would give you a firm diagnosis. You actually saw bones that would be porous and poorly formed.

This changed after Merck developed a terrible drug called Fosamax to treat osteoporosis. It doesn't really work and has been linked to all kinds of side effects, including fractures to the thighbone[10]—the very sort of thing you'd think it would help prevent—and osteonecrosis (bone death) of the jaw.[11] But in the beginning, the problem was that there weren't enough people being diagnosed with osteoporosis. So Merck hired a marketing expert to change that. A conference was convened in Rome in 1992, sponsored by drug companies, during which medical experts, if you want to call them that, got together and redefined the diagnostic criteria for osteoporosis. It would henceforth be the loss of bone mineral density that would be the diagnostic criteria.[12]

The problem with that is that all people lose bone mineral density as they age, particularly women. Women have very strong skeletons because they need strong bones for childbearing; when we're past our childbearing years, we lose bone density. I'm not planning on carrying any more children, so my bones don't have to be as strong as they were when I was twenty-eight. Merck succeeded in developing diagnostic criteria that would eventually include everybody. In a process called disease-mongering, the definition of a disease is expanded so that more and more people will qualify and get treatment. The other thing that happened at this meeting was that they picked an arbitrary amount of bone mineral density loss that was not based on any science. The question came up: What about people on the other side of the arbitrary line who aren't yet qualified for osteoporosis but are getting close? So they made up the mythical disease called osteopenia. Merck, being the ever-accommodating company, actually developed a lower dose of Fosamax to treat those people who had the mythical condition that was considered a precursor to the even worse mythical condition.

GM: So osteopenia is simply less loss of bone mineral density than osteoporosis?

PP: Yes. Osteopenia is a stepping-stone. You're told, once you're diagnosed with this mythical disease, that if you don't do something about it, you're going to progress to the next level of mythical disease.

GM: So there are no symptoms? Osteopenia is merely a way station, like purgatory?

PP: Except that I think there's probably more scientific proof of purgatory.

GM: But don't we live in a nation of elderly people falling down and fracturing themselves? Is that just natural or is something wrong?

PP: Well, first of all, let me make what sounds like an obvious, asinine statement: the number-one cause of fractures is falling. But why do people fall? They fall because they're frail, on drugs, or have poor balance and coordination. People who haven't exercised become frail. My mother hasn't exercised since 1956, so it's not surprising that she's terribly frail. Of course, we're further frightened by the idea that once these falls happen and bones are broken, these people often become bedridden and then die; we're told it's the hip fracture that killed them. Well, it isn't the fracture that killed them; it's the poor health and the drugs they were taking that caused the fall in the first place. They're fracturing bones because of the trajectory of the fall in many instances. I'm not saying that nobody has osteoporosis; we see people in here who have it, but I'm saying the vast majority of people who think they have it, don't. These Dexa scans to determine bone density are very unreliable.[13] Many, many health agencies in other countries have said that there's no relationship between bone mineral density and fracture risk and that the Dexa scan tells us nothing.

GM: But you do acknowledge that some people have osteoporosis, meaning some people have very low bone density?

PP: Right.

GM: And is the cause related to diet, or is it just genetics?

PP: First, it's lifestyle as it relates to exercise, or the lack thereof. It can also be diet related as it pertains to developing a GI disorder, like inflammatory bowel diseases, where you're not absorbing nutrients. The other cause is a condition called metabolic acidosis, in which you eat animal foods, highly processed foods, or foods with a high sulfur content—animal protein is highly sulfuric— and these sulfur compounds increase the acid load in the body, necessitating the withdrawal of calcium from the bones in order for the body to maintain proper pH.

GM: And the calcium is eliminated through the process of urination?

53

PP: Yes, you literally pee out your calcium. People drink milk because it allegedly builds strong bones due to its calcium, but in fact the high sulfuric protein content of milk winds up costing the body calcium; that's why the highest rates of osteoporosis are in countries with the highest dairy intake.[14]

GM: Have there been any studies that have proved this dynamic of metabolic acidosis?

PP: Yes, absolutely.[15,16,17,18] A meta-analysis of eighteen separate studies published on bone health found that fourteen of them, or about 78 percent, supported the idea that low-acid eating improves bone health.[19] So the preponderance of the evidence shows that eating animal foods causes the body to use calcium drawn from the bones to buffer the acid in order for the body to maintain blood pH within a very narrow range. We can measure how much calcium somebody takes in; it's quantifiable. We can also measure how much you urinate; that's also quantifiable. If you're excreting more than you're taking in, it's coming from somewhere.

GM: What brings on acid reflux?

PP: Diet and lifestyle. It's related to several things, but one is weight. Overweight people tend to have acid reflux because the sheer force of their weight sometimes weakens the esophageal sphincter, particularly when they are lying down. Overeating is another cause. Eating large meals that expand the stomach way beyond its capacity contributes to it. Constipation also contributes to it because all that straining pushes the diaphragm up and puts pressure on the esophageal sphincter. Certain foods, which would include alcohol, caffeine, and foods high in fat, tend to aggravate acid reflux. What's amazing is that within a fairly short period of time, there's generally relief from acid reflux as soon as people stop eating a terrible diet.

GM: Let's move on to multiple sclerosis (MS). Genes or diet or something else?

PP: MS is definitely diet, particularly saturated fat and dairy intake. Lifestyle can also be a factor in terms of stress, which can exacerbate MS, but diet is the primary culprit.

GM: MS can actually be caused by diet?

PP: Yes, absolutely.

GM: Where is the evidence for that?

PP: Even as far back as the 1940s, there was evidence that diet played a role. For example, in areas of the world where fat consumption was higher (more than one hundred grams per day), the incidence of multiple sclerosis was higher, too. In areas where fat consumption was less than fifty grams per day, the incidence of multiple sclerosis was lower.[20] Studies in Norway confirmed this: in areas of the country where fat consumption was higher, the incidence of MS was higher, and saturated fat was the most harmful.[21] But I think the most compelling evidence we have comes from Dr. Roy Swank, who developed a theory sixty years ago stating that there were certain causes of multiple sclerosis, one of which was poor diet that eventually compromised the blood/ brain barrier and the intestinal barrier. It would take a long time to explain the mechanism of action, but the bottom line for him was to test his theory by placing thirty-four patients on a low-fat diet, very low saturated fat. The results were astounding.[22]

Some of Dr. Swank's patients were compliant and others were not. He categorized his patients based on their fat consumption—"good dieters" consumed less than twenty grams per day of saturated fat; "bad dieters" consumed more than twenty grams per day. Patients in the group consuming less than twenty grams of saturated fat per day fared significantly better than the group eating more saturated fat. For those who ate a low-saturated fat diet, "about 95% [. . .] remained only mildly disabled for approximately 30 years." Eighty percent of the patients who consumed more saturated fat died of MS.[23] Dr. Swank published several articles in medical journals documenting his results.[24, 25, 26] He duplicated those results on thousands of additional patients and showed that patients on a low-fat diet with a minimal amount of animal foods basically remained asymptomatic. The exacerbation rate—exacerbations are what they call these flare-ups that MS patients experience—went down by 95 percent and stayed that way in compliant patients.

GM: Dr. McDougall is doing a similar study now.

PP: He is. His diet—and I learned about diet and MS from Dr. McDougall—is a little bit different from Dr. Swank's: no animal foods, no low-fat dairy, no oils. According to Dr. McDougall, Dr. Swank acknowledged before he died that the inclusion of oils had no therapeutic value. He thought it might make people more compliant on the diet, but he didn't attribute his success to the inclusion of oil. So Dr. McDougall's diet is lower in fat. And the results are even better. It's amazing, and we see that here, too. It's complete regression of the disease, so much so that I would call it a reversal of the disease, especially in patients who adopt the diet in the early stages of the disease. People say, "How can you make that claim?" Well, there are two things that are common to MS patients: an intolerance of heat and a lack of stamina or endurance. We have Wellness Forum members with MS who are doing bike rides for three hundred miles, taking hot yoga classes in a 105 degree room. They don't take any drugs and have absolutely no symptoms. At this point in time we would pronounce them former MS patients.

GM: So they have no symptoms?

PP: None.

GM: Is there any marker for the disease other than its symptoms?

PP: In the early stages, no. That's what makes diagnosis really difficult. Most patients start with what we call "relapsing-remitting MS," which means that they get symptoms and then they go away. Then a few weeks later they get symptoms and then they go away and the symptoms change. The doctors will say, "I can't find anything wrong with you," and sometimes send them to a psychiatrist. They'll even take spinal taps; nothing shows anything so "maybe you've got a mental problem," they are told. Doctors send them to a psychiatrist instead of telling them to improve their diet. They can go for a really long time without a firm diagnosis. Eventually you can see, through proper imaging, what looks like plaques or lesions in different areas of the central nervous system. There are some tests, a flicker fusion vision test, and some various tests you can do to test reflexes that sometimes give you a pretty definitive diagnosis, but in the early stages, there is no definitive diagnosis.

GM: What about influenza? Does it have any cause other than contagion?

PP: Well, it is contagious, but whether or not you get it, and how severe it is, depends upon your health status. About five years ago, one of the most virulent strains of flu ran through Columbus, Ohio, that I can remember in my entire life. It was heinous. I belong to a lot of groups, and people were missing work for three weeks at a time; we were having meetings with half of the people there. One school closed for a couple days because there were so many kids sick. It was bad. And at first, none of us got sick here at The Wellness Forum, even though we're exposed to sick people every day in this office. Then one day I woke up around four in the morning (I'm an early riser), and I was as sick as a dog. I was sick for maybe four or five hours, and then it went away. I was just tired, so I took a nice nap and came into the office around one or two and made it a short day. By the next day, I was back to normal.

Well, sure enough, the next day Gary, our general manager, woke up with the flu. He had it for about four or five hours, came in later in the afternoon, and was fine afterward. One by one, it cycled through the office. We all actually got it, but nobody missed more than a half a day of work because of it. I think many times I don't get what's going around because I'm a very uninviting host for disease. And if I do get it, or somebody around here gets something, it's usually a nonevent. Nobody here misses work much for anything, and we're exposed to more sickness than most people.

GM: My old man died of Parkinson's. Is it genetic?

PP: Even if there are some genetic predispositions to it, and there may well be, I think that definitely diet and lifestyle play a significant role. Chemical exposure may be involved as well; we just don't know. The sad part is that by the time somebody has full-blown Parkinson's, we don't usually see diet and lifestyle reversing it. What we do see is that it'll stop or slow its progression, which can be a blessing for the person who has Parkinson's and anybody caring for that person, but we don't normally see the regression that you see in MS and some of these other conditions.

GM: Have you been able to slow or stop its progression?

PP: Both, depending on how bad our clients are when they become members and start eating a plant-based diet. Sometimes we get people in such late stages that all we can do is slow it. Again, it's not the way I wish it were, but it's better than nothing. As these people degenerate, they lose their ability to communicate, or to do anything for themselves; they become tremendous burdens on their families, so even a minor reduction in the rate of its progression can make a big difference.

GM: Rheumatoid arthritis?

PP: It's almost always diet and lifestyle related, and is particularly related to the consumption of animal foods.

GM: And that's not commonly accepted wisdom, either?

PP: Oh, no. The conventional wisdom is wrong, but as I said, it's not easy to change the conventional wisdom of people in this country, including health professionals.

GM: Does genetics play a role in rheumatoid arthritis?

PP: Yes. Genetics can make you predisposed. I am positive I am predisposed. I am positive I could make myself have it in a very short time, particularly at my current age. But I don't eat like my mother, my grandmother, or the other members of my family who have this dreadful disease.

GM: What are the causes of asthma?

PP: Well, there are a lot of things that can cause asthma. There are environmental triggers and dietary triggers for sure, dairy being one of the most common.[27, 28] Dehydration is a factor;[29] a lot of kids are not very good water drinkers, so that has an impact. Poor GI health contributes; people who have screwed-up GI tracts often have respiratory disorders, including allergies and asthma. We see a lot of asthma in children, which is related to many factors, including poor gut ecology due to constipation; treatment with antibiotics; and, in some situations, even vaccinations. Their guts are not very healthy and their immune systems are overstimulated. The overuse of antibiotics due to chronic infection compromises the health of their GI tracts and contributes to it as well. Respiratory toxins aggravate the situation.

Asthma tends to get better in kids if you take the dairy out of the diet, get the kid drinking enough water, put him or her on a program of dietary excellence (a whole foods, plant-based diet), and add some probiotic supplements. Generally speaking, it improves to the point where they often don't even have to use an inhaler for exercise. In older people who've had it for a long time, it takes longer to get better, but they follow the same protocol with the addition of supplements like quercetin. I recommend sea salt as a natural antihistamine. I don't recommend against salt consumption for most people, as you know, so we recommend sea salt as an antihistamine, more so in adults than kids.

GM: So how does the salt work—how much do people have to consume?

PP: We use it therapeutically; how it is used and the dose depend on the age of the individual.

Even in those cases where asthma or environmental allergies don't entirely go away, with a change in diet, people can become a lot more comfortable and reduce their dependence on antihistamines and medications.

GM: It isn't very intuitive that the GI tract would have something to do with a respiratory disease.

PP: There are a number of connections between asthma and GI function, including reflux and beneficial bacteria in the GI tract. Reflux contributes to asthma, because the acid is inhaled through the back of the throat, burns the bronchial tubes, and causes symptoms of asthma.[30, 31]

Beneficial bacteria in the GI tract are very important in regulating immune function. It is compromised by taking antibiotics, steroids, and other drugs, as well as by constipation and inflammatory bowel diseases. When enough beneficial bacteria are destroyed, leaky gut can result, allowing whole-food particles to enter the bloodstream, leading to compromised or overactive immunity, allergic responses to foods, and systemic inflammation. An overactive immune system and systemic inflammation can contribute to the development of asthma.

GM: What causes gallstones?

PP: It's definitely diet related. Gallstones are made of cholesterol in nearly all cases. People end up with gallstones from eating a high-fat, animal-protein diet. Unfortunately, one problem we have in medicine today is the overriding view by a lot of doctors that body parts are disposable. "Oh, if it's bothering you, we'll just take it out."

GM: So the gallbladder goes.

61

PP: The gallbladder goes, or maybe the spleen or the appendix go. I happen to think we have these body parts for a reason and we should work hard to preserve them. Unless the disease has progressed to the place where it's horrific, most people who change to the diet we're promoting would experience relief from the pain associated with gallstones and gallbladder disease. As long as they're compliant, they're fine. I've had members who say, "I eat one high-fat meal and I'm miserable," and I tell them, "Good, that's a good way to keep you on the straight and narrow. We don't have to worry so much about you because you have an instant adverse effect from straying."

It's not unusual, of course, for people to have their gallbladder removed. Then they continue their dietary habits and find out they're still just as uncomfortable because all of the fat and animal protein that they're eating is so detrimental to their health. They're usually fairly distressed to find out that some of their discomfort is coming from bile acids dripping right into the colon, which is why they still feel nauseous and sick. And the presence of bile acids in the colon increases their risk of colon cancer substantially. They were promised instantaneous relief from their discomfort; however, they end up with long-term increased risk of colon cancer and no relief from their symptoms.[32] I would say that that probably happens 35 or 40 percent of the time following gallbladder removal.

GM: So having your gallbladder removed increases your risk of colon cancer?

PP: Yes. And we all acknowledge that there are situations where the gallbladder is just so diseased that you have to take it out, but doctors tend to be really cavalier about removing body parts. I think it's always worthwhile to see if a change in diet, if somebody's willing to do it, affects the situation. Sometimes it happens so quickly—I'm talking about a matter of days—that someone calls his doctor and says, "That surgery I had scheduled for next Friday? I don't need to do it now because I'm feeling much better."

GM: Have you had Wellness Forum members who did that?

PP: Yes. I've also had members who have had their gallbladder taken out. The unfortunate reality is that what we want as human beings, from both the doctor's perspective and the patient's perspective, is resolution. The doctor and the patient want it resolved, and there's something satisfying about just taking it out. The disease is gone. It's over with, and we can just put it behind us. That's not really the case, but that's the perception a lot of people have that lead them to engage in, or consent to, risky medical practices.

GM: So if somebody has a diseased gallbladder, riddled with gallstones, and then he adopts the correct diet, will those gallstones just dissolve?

PP: Sometimes they will, but usually they just stop causing problems. If the gallstones get caught in the duct, that's when you may have to do something surgically, but not always.

GM: And what about kidney stones?

PP: Well, that's the result of several factors. The first is increased calcium concentration, which comes about from the high calcium intake that people in this country have been convinced is necessary. We have a lot of people taking calcium supplements and, of course, consuming cow's milk. The other cause of high calcium levels is the release of calcium from the bones to buffer acidity, the metabolic acidosis that results from consuming a lot of protein, fat, refined foods, caffeine, alcohol, etc. Combine the high calcium levels with dehydration, and our poor little kidneys are forced to concentrate more and more waste with less and less fluid. You can end up with some kidney stones. They can become a thing of the past, even for people who have a lot of them, if they just start drinking enough filtered water every day and eating a healthy, whole foods, plant-based diet.

GM: How many glasses of filtered water?

PP: I like for people to drink sixty-four ounces of water a day as a base. That's for adults. Children should drink half their weight in ounces. And then you have to compensate for activities. Yesterday I ran, went to the gym, taught a hot yoga class, and then took a hot sweatbox class, so I probably had three gallons of water to compensate.

I've heard people insist that if you eat the right diet, you don't need to drink water. I disagree. We need to remember that thirst is not an adequate or reliable indicator of the need for water. There are a couple of reasons for that. One is that we salivate when we eat, which disguises the thirst response. The second is that our bodies adapt to dehydration. Eventually, just as if you don't eat long enough, you don't feel hungry anymore, if you don't drink water for a long enough time, you learn to live with dehydration and not necessarily feel thirsty. As evidence, consider the number of people who end up hospitalized for dehydration every year, in perfectly ordinary circumstances, when they could easily have reached for a drink of water.

One of the smartest people I know runs a multimillion-dollar company here in Columbus. A couple of years ago, at a meeting in New York, he passed out on the floor. They took him to the hospital; he was just dehydrated. Now, I'm sure that if this very smart, educated, wealthy guy thought that he was thirsty, he would have reached for something to drink. To insist that all of this would just be remedied if we would drink just when we're thirsty and not worry about it the rest of the time is to miss the lesson in incidences like this, which are not uncommon.

GM: Food poisoning is obviously a dietary issue, but is there one type of diet that makes you less likely to get food poisoning than another?

PP: One way you can avoid food poisoning is to avoid chicken, fish, pork, beef, and the other foods that are more likely to give you food poisoning. The second thing is that healthy people, even exposed to a pathogen, often don't have any response to it. So if you've got really well-established colonies of beneficial bacteria in your system, even exposure to a pathogen may not make any difference. Generally, food poisoning results from consuming animal foods, with some rare exceptions like the one that happened a few years ago when spinach was contaminated by animals near the farm. The spinach was not the cause of the food poisoning; it was the nearby environmental abusers, like cattle ranches, causing the food poisoning.

GM: Yeah, it always bugs me when the news media reports some scare, like E. coli in lettuce, without noting animal agriculture as a likely cause. They make it sound like it's normal, like some lettuce from a bad seed just grows into pathological lettuce.

PP: I have no idea what they're thinking, but our best defense in any case remains maintaining colonies of beneficial bacteria, while limiting or eliminating the animal foods that generally expose us to the harmful bacteria.

GM: Does eating soy yogurt help a person get those healthy bacteria? How do you get the healthy bacteria?

PP: Well, first of all, you're born with it. You acquire it during vaginal delivery.[33] One problem we have is the overuse of Caesarean deliveries, most of them unnecessary. The baby's normal way of acquiring beneficial bacteria, which is moving through the birth canal, isn't happening as frequently, so the baby is acquiring bacteria from the hospital environment, which impairs the child.

Another way that the baby develops beneficial bacteria is through breast-feeding.[34] So a Caesarean-born, bottle-fed baby has an automatic disadvantage. That child is at a disadvantage for the rest of her life. That doesn't mean bad things are going to happen; it means they are more likely to happen. But let's just say that a baby is vaginally born, is breast-fed, and has healthy bacteria. That child will be fine unless she does something to destroy it, like take antibiotics or birth control pills, develop constipation, irritable bowel or inflammatory bowel conditions, or celiac disease. Those kinds of conditions impact the beneficial bacteria in the GI tract. If you've had any of those things happen, you need to take strong, pharmaceutical-grade probiotics in order to fix it.

GM: Well, most Americans have taken an antibiotic now and then.

PP: Right, and this is something I get angry about. One hundred percent of all doctors surveyed will tell you that taking an antibiotic destroys beneficial bacteria. Yet in any metropolitan area, you can count on one hand the number of doctors who put their patients on probiotics to compensate for the destruction of the antibiotic regimen. We have a lot of folks out there who have taken not just one antibiotic regimen but twenty-five or thirty of them in their lifetime and never fixed the damage. They need good pharmaceutical-grade probiotics. You're not going to replenish a destroyed colony by eating yogurt of any type. There aren't enough of the critters in the yogurt to establish the colonies. Eating soy yogurt may help a little; people claim benefits from consuming probiotic-laced products, but they don't really grow colonies. You get some temporary relief from the symptoms, but you don't resolve the underlying issue.

Having a healthy colony of beneficial bacteria is crucial for your immune function, your ability to absorb nutrients from food, and your ability to keep the intestinal barrier healthy so that partially digested food and other pathogens and bacteria don't get into the bloodstream.

GM: And these pharmaceutical-grade probiotics, can you get them in health food stores?

PP: You can get better ones from a doctor or another knowledgeable practitioner. A lot of the best companies don't sell their products in health food stores for a couple of reasons. First of all, some people can hurt themselves with these products. For example, if a person with active Crohn's disease walked into a store, bought a really strong product, and took it home, he might end up in the hospital as a result of taking it. It could increase their diarrhea considerably, and a Crohn's patient definitely doesn't need more diarrhea. I found that the best probiotics manufacturers sell their products through practitioners rather than through health food stores.

GM: Let's discuss the causes of irritable bowel syndrome, ulcerative colitis, and Crohn's disease.

PP: Absolutely diet and lifestyle. For some people, there's also a psychological component in the case of irritable bowel; while the syndrome is biological in nature, there is some evidence that it can be brought about by psychological factors.[35]

There are two ways in which our thoughts and emotions can impact GI health. The first is that we actually have a nervous system in our GI tract called the enteric nervous system that operates independent of our autonomic and central nervous systems. This is what causes you to have a "gut feeling" about something. This is what causes you to have diarrhea or a stomach ache in response to stress or something of that nature. Butterflies in your stomach are your enteric nervous system acting up a bit. Also, there are certain psychological profiles of people who are more inclined to develop and maintain irritable bowel, even when you do all the right things to fix it. They continue to have it, sometimes because they get secondary gain from hanging on to the disease. Some of these people had trauma or were rewarded for sickness as children. They got excused from going to school if they had a tummy ache. Or they got excused from dinner and were given ice cream instead. So some people learn secondary gain from using gastrointestinal disorders of an undefined nature and those people grow up sometimes to have irritable bowel syndrome. There's a little bit more of a complex causation with irritable bowel than with other ailments. On the other hand, I can say with a great deal of confidence that inflammatory bowel diseases are at base the result of diet and lifestyle choices.

GM: Is dairy one of the main culprits?

PP: Dairy is a big culprit. Animal foods are also a culprit, as are high-gluten foods: barley, rye, oats, and wheat.

GM: Now you're talking about good, healthy, vegan foods that could cause trouble.

PP: Nuts are good foods, too, but if you go into anaphylactic shock when you eat them, you wouldn't say they're particularly good for you. High-gluten foods are really deadly for these people. They have to maintain complete abstinence from barley, rye, oats, and wheat in order to maintain the complete remission from their disease. The good news is that people with inflammatory bowel diseases who follow the dietary recommendations we give them—a low-fat, plant-based diet, which is phased in over time—achieve excellent results.[36]

GM: And that's the next malady I was going to ask you about: celiac disease.

PP: Celiac disease has a genetic predisposition. I don't think somebody eats her way into celiac disease. There is some evidence that a virus or precipitating events can contribute to it. You have to do a couple of things to recover from celiac disease. One is to stop consuming any gluten; you eliminate any exposure to gluten at all, including tiny amounts of gluten as an ingredient in soy sauce and things of that nature. You have to be very diligent about it. You also take probiotics to restore the beneficial bacteria that's been destroyed. Many people have been undiagnosed for years, so they present with considerable destruction to the GI tract. If they spend a long time taking a high-grade probiotic product, they can restore their health if they eat the right diet and abstain from all gluten products.

GM: Do you advocate blood tests to determine if someone has celiac disease?

PP: The blood test is not always definitive. The most definitive test is to take a biopsy and look at the tissue; if all the little villi are destroyed, then the person is a celiac patient. But I don't think we have to go that far. If someone has a family history of celiac disease and has gotten better since giving up gluten, that's enough evidence in many cases. Somebody asked me during a class why doctors subject these patients to a lot of these tests. I said, "Well, some people show up with a very big disadvantage when they arrive in a doctor's office or a hospital; it's called "good insurance." One of the worst things you can have if you're at a facility where they like to do testing is good insurance. If they know it's going to be paid for, they'll subject you to as much of it as can possibly be arranged.

GM: We haven't talked about one of the leading causes of death in America, which is iatrogenic death, or death caused by medical treatment.

PP: The numbers are astounding.

GM: And when I research it, I see wildly varying estimates. Wikipedia comes up with a figure of 225,000 deaths per year; critics of the American medical system will estimate more like 800,000 or 900,000 deaths per year.

PP: Dr. T. Colin Campbell and Dr. McDougall are among those critics.

GM: It's obviously hard to know exactly what the correct figure is because so many people, especially older people, whose death may be brought on by a medication, never have that fact determined in court, and their death certificates don't reflect that cause.

PP: Well, I think the problem's getting worse. I can just tell you from my own experience, people who join The Wellness Forum are often as sick from medical care as they are from whatever was ailing them when they first started receiving medical care. Or they were perfectly healthy people who were treated for mythical diseases like osteoporosis or carcinoma in situ and become sick patients as the result of being treated for diseases they never had. In terms of what the actual numbers are, the most reliable numbers I've seen come from sources like Shannon Brownlee's book, *Overtreated*,[37] a well-referenced book on the topic. Even the *Journal of the American Medical Association* has published articles showing that between 230,000 and 284,000 deaths per year result from medical treatment. This does not include adverse effects from medication that result in sickness or disability, which are estimated to result in 116 million extra physician visits, 77 million extra prescriptions, 17 million emergency department visits, 8 million hospitalizations, 3 million long-term admissions, 199,000 additional deaths, and $77 billion in extra costs (equivalent to the total cost of taking care of patients with diabetes).[38] It's generally accepted that dying from medical treatment is the third- or fourth-leading cause of death in this country; at least a few hundred thousand or potentially more people die every year directly as a result of the treatment that they receive.

Now, I'll mitigate that frightening statistic somewhat. Some of the people who die from medical treatment were really sick and decrepit when they entered the hospital; while they received treatment that may have been useless and may have sped up their death, they were going to die anyway. That said, there's still an atrocious amount of death from medical treatment arising from the treatment of conditions that patients don't really have. From overmedication or unnecessary surgery. From suicides brought on by useless antidepressant and antianxiety drugs. Overall, it's certainly one of the leading causes of death in the country. That's why Dr. McDougall says, "Stay away from doctors; they'll kill you."

GM: Pam, having reviewed now a significant list of diseases and ailments, what's revealed to me is the sweeping and I'd say revolutionary nature of your work. Under standard medical care, a very sick patient presenting with heart disease, diabetes, high blood pressure, acid reflux, and irritable bowel syndrome would spend his days shuttling between his cardiologist, gastroenterologist, and otolaryngologist, getting different medications or interventions for each condition. Then he'd have to hope that his medications don't interact in a dangerous way. He'd find himself on a slippery slope to doom. And there are millions of Americans who live that way, if you could call it living. Now, you would argue that all these conditions are essentially expressions of the same disease that is the Western diet, and that the remedy for all the conditions is essentially the same: a low-fat, plant-based diet. With this diet, it's quite possible no medications would be needed at all, for almost any condition.

PP: That's exactly right.

GM: Unfortunately, there are only a few places in America that take this very simple and comprehensive approach to disease, most notably Dr. McDougall's practice in Santa Rosa, California, and your own Wellness Forum based in Columbus, Ohio.

PP: That's why we need to get the word out.

GM: Since food is actually the leading cause of disease, let's get very specific now about different types of food. What's wrong, for example, with fish?

PP: There's a misperception that fish is a healthier form of animal food when, in fact, it's actually higher in fat than many animal foods. The misperception causes people to replace red meat with fish and feel that they have improved their health when they really haven't. If they eat too much fish, they may have actually made things worse because of the high fat content.

GM: But we've heard so often that it's healthy fat; it's full of omega fatty acids.

PP: I think that there isn't any such thing as healthy fat beyond a certain percentage in the diet. The idea is to eat a very low-fat diet: 15 percent at the upper end and 9 to 11 percent at the lower end for people who have coronary artery disease, obesity, and certain other conditions. So when more than 50 percent of the calories in salmon are from fat, you can't eat a whole lot of that and keep yourself within that range.

GM: Is the fat from fish better than the fat from beef?

PP: If you're crossing that 15 percent line, I don't think it makes any difference at all. And while many claim that fish is somehow protective, there have been some interesting studies on Japanese men that show that the more fish they eat, the higher the incidence of prostate cancer.[39] At a certain point, you cross that threshold in terms of the allowable amounts of animal protein and fat; fish becomes just another flesh food, and bad things start to happen. There are also the dangers presented by mercury and other toxins in fish. At the end of the day, the source of that animal fat and protein doesn't make much difference; it doesn't matter if you're getting it from eggs, fish, chicken, turkey, pork—it's really all the same thing.

GM: We've all heard studies reported in the news that fish allegedly protects the heart. My theory is that when they do these studies and they compare fish eaters to beef eaters, it's possible that salmon is marginally less bad for the heart than beef. People have better outcomes in terms of sudden cardiac death with fish than beef, but they've never done a study comparing fish eaters to vegans.

PP: Right. But there's another complication, too. There are some studies that show that eating fish and or taking fish oil capsules will raise HDL, or "good cholesterol," levels, which is one reason it's touted as being protective. But that doesn't make any difference. In other words, we don't really have any evidence showing that higher HDL levels are the key to better cardiovascular health. And, in fact, two drugs never made it to market, very promising drugs, not by my definition, but by the definition of drug companies and the traditional cardiology profession. These two drugs, dalcetrapib, which was developed by Roche, and torcetrapib, which was developed by Pfizer, were designed to elevate HDL cholesterol; both did that quite well. The one little problem was that the people with the higher HDL levels were dying off faster than the people with lower HDL levels, so those drugs never came to market. The concern with the ratio of HDL to LDL is completely misplaced.[40]

GM: So have doctors across America misunderstood this, or have they all been misled? How did this happen?

PP: It's a fundamental misunderstanding about the role of HDL, which is to help to clear the bad cholesterol from the bloodstream. As your LDL levels ratchet down, which they do on a low-fat, plant-based diet, the need for HDL will also ratchet down. If you look at populations like the Tarahumara of northwestern Mexico, who typically have very, very low cholesterol levels, they also have low HDL levels. I love Dr. Caldwell Esselstyn's line; he says "the HDL levels of the Tarahumara Indians would make the average cardiologist in the United States apoplectic." Why? Because they would be certain that it would be deadly. We're talking about HDL levels in the range of fourteen to twenty-four milligrams per deciliters, which is very, very low.[41] The Tarahumara eat a plant-based diet centered around corn and have a low incidence of heart disease.

GM: We've talked about fish. What do you think about chicken?

PP: I sometimes refer to the strategy of replacing one bad food with another as rearranging the deck chairs on the *Titanic*. Chicken is just another animal food, and a particularly filthy one at that. It's another food that has a face and a mother, which is how we define animal food around here. The same detrimental effect that we would expect to experience by consuming too much beef in our diets, we'll see with too much chicken in the diet. We've got to stop imagining that there's some animal out there that's really healthy to consume. We've got to understand that if animal foods are consumed more than two to three times per week, and even that may be too much for some people, we're going to have problems; it really doesn't much matter what animal we pick. Chicken, even white meat chicken, is high in fat. Again, it's extraordinarily difficult if this is going to be part of the daily fare to keep fat consumption in line.

And it's not just the excessive fat that's a problem. There's no fiber. There are no phytochemicals and antioxidants. When people develop cancer, what really is going on, on a certain level, is that cancer promoters have outnumbered the anticancer agents in the diet. We have to consider the anticancer properties of food, the phytochemicals like indole-3-carbinol that we see in, for example, cruciferous vegetables. Well, chicken doesn't contain those, or any other antioxidants. It offers absolutely no protection, and that's why I say if it rises above the level of condiment in the diet, it's deadly. There are no "better" animal foods. When we start talking about grass-fed beef and organic beef and organic chicken and those sorts of things, we're still talking about a product that has no fiber, no phytochemicals, no antioxidants, and is high in fat. Yes, we avoid some of the hormones, steroids, and antibiotics that are given to conventionally raised animals, but the amino acid chains that make up those animal foods are exactly the same, and they're just as cancer promoting at a certain concentration in the diet. All the evidence points in the same direction: you should not consume much of this stuff, or any of it at all. My preference is none at all.

GM: I like to look at it this way: carbohydrate is the most efficient fuel for the human body.

PP: Right. And when the body is forced to use fat or protein for fuel, it'll do it, but it's a very cumbersome process; it's very stressful and quite toxic to the body to do that.

GM: So we know that carbohydrate is the natural fuel for the human body and we know that fiber is necessary and health promoting to the human body. Yet we look at these flesh foods and they have no fiber and no carbohydrates. It strikes me as a clue that they're not human foods.

PP: Right. These are not the foods we were designed to live on. Our intestinal tracts are long. We need a lot of fiber to push food through the system, and the primary enzyme that's secreted in your saliva is amylase, which is an enzyme that breaks down starch. We could anatomically take a little tour through the digestive system, starting with what happens when food enters the mouth, and make a strong case for our design being geared toward consuming plant food.

GM: Which brings us to another high-fat, high-protein, zero-fiber, low-carbohydrate animal food: dairy.

PP: I think that's the most toxic of all. When I give lectures, I get asked, "If I were going to do one thing and one thing only, what would you suggest I do?" Well, one change alone won't do the trick if you're eating the standard American diet. But if you're going to make an important first step that would improve your health, get the dairy out of the diet. Dairy products have no upside. On the downside, dairy proteins have been linked to asthma, allergies, chronic constipation, chronic ear infections in children,[42, 43] multiple sclerosis,[44] autoimmune diseases, breast cancer, prostate cancer,[45] and osteoporosis.[46] The likelihood that a genetically susceptible child consuming dairy products will develop juvenile diabetes is actually greater than the likelihood of a smoker developing lung cancer.[47, 48, 49] That's kind of hard to wrap your arms around when you think about it, particularly since our government actually promotes the consumption of dairy products by children.

GM: People who follow the federal dietary guidelines, the ever-changing pyramids and plates that the United States Department of Agriculture (USDA) spends untold millions revising, believe they're eating a balanced diet. Are they so wrong in believing that their diet of fruit and vegetables and grains on the one hand, and dairy and eggs and meat on the other hand, is at least balanced?

PP: Only in the sense that it can lead to a balanced need for various types of medical interventions. Here's something I've observed: a family of four people sits down to eat dinner in a restaurant and there's absolutely nothing on the table they're eating that I would put in my mouth. You have one person eating a cheeseburger and fries. The next is eating chicken and cheese quesadillas. And the next one is having a spinach quiche. The last one is having a turkey sandwich. They're all drinking sodas and lemonade. This is the whole family's dinner. It would probably be heartily endorsed by the USDA and there's not a single worthwhile, nutritious thing on the table. They just have no idea that the meal they just spent fifty or sixty bucks on is worth nothing nutritionally. "Oh, cheese is good for your bones, the chicken is lower in fat than the beef, and the fries must be better because they're housemade. Oh, and it's Diet Coke." They use all this ridiculous criteria to justify the choice of these foods and believe that they're doing reasonably well, but it's all just horrible.

GM: Beyond animal foods, there are other sins in the standard American diet.

PP: There's the fat content in general, but what makes it really horrendous are the oils; people cook with oils, packaged foods and baked goods contain oil, salad dressings are full of oil, and restaurants overuse it. So people consume enormous amounts of oil and fat in the diet. And enormous amounts of plain junk foods.

GM: What about sugar and sweets?

PP: Well, I always tell people that we can't vilify individual constituents because it's the pattern that makes the difference, but sugar is just empty calories and is also addictive. I don't know very many people—I can think of a handful—who can be around sweets without eating them. I personally don't like those people. I'm very envious of them because if it's in front of me, I want to eat it. Dr. Neal Barnard, in his book *Breaking the Food Seduction*, writes that there are studies that have shown that the effect of sugar on the dopamine receptors of the brain is very similar to the effect of drugs like heroin and cocaine on those dopamine receptors. Most people don't understand when they buy this stuff at the store that it has a highly addictive quality and that they're going to want more and more of it.

Not only do sweets not provide any nutritive value, and one could argue that they're destructive to health in terms of elevating blood sugar levels and suppressing immune function, but they displace healthy foods in the diet. If someone eats eight hundred calories' worth of cookies and brownies in a day, that's eight hundred calories that aren't going into sweet potatoes and vegetables and rice and other foods that would actually have some protective value.

The other thing to remember is that these refined sugary foods elevate triglycerides. And triglycerides are blood fats waiting to cause mischief. Triglycerides and cholesterol will go down when you get rid of all that refined and processed sugar-filled stuff.

GM: Now, is there anything wrong with buying a box of crackers, whether it's something like Ritz crackers, or even crackers you might see in a health food store made with whole wheat flour and organic sesame seeds and so forth?

PP: There's definitely something wrong with the Ritz crackers. The top ingredients for your regular, store-bought cracker brands, the ones that most people would know about, are sugar, white flour, and some type of fat. This is just absolutely junk food. There's no nutritive value to it; you don't want to buy it. When it comes to crackers in a health food store, you can find a few that don't contain oil. However, any type of processed food like that is going to be calorie-dense. You really don't want to be filling your diet with calorie-dense food.

I don't completely abstain from eating crackers, but they're not a staple of my diet. I like fat-free hummus; I use it for vegetable wraps, but I also like to eat it as a dip. Now most people would dip crackers in it; I dip mushroom slices, sliced cucumbers, carrots, and things like that in the hummus. They're much better for you than crackers. If I were having a party this weekend, I might have some crackers, but I'm working alone this weekend, so I'll be dipping my mushroom slices in the hummus.

GM: Okay, let's talk about fatty plant foods. Let's assume you're eating these foods in their whole state. Avocado—anything wrong with that?

PP: Well, there's nothing wrong with any of these foods for a relatively healthy person. Avocados, nuts, seeds, olives—I love them. What I tell people is that they don't want to be going out of their way to consume them, though, because they can end up eating a diet that's quite high in fat with those foods. Our Chef Del is a good example. On a totally vegan diet, he ate himself to 475 pounds.

GM: What the heck was he eating?

PP: High-fat plant foods, fried food, baked goods . . . Del used to eat lots of avocados and almonds by the handful. Now he's lost half of himself. I want to make that clear; he's done a great job since he's been here. So my rule is that I eat these fatty plant foods when they occur in a dish, but I don't go out of my way to eat them. A restaurant near my house makes black bean wraps and the chef puts slices of avocado in them; I eat that. We have a dish here called vegetable byriani that has almonds in it; I eat that. But I don't buy avocados at the store and put them on all of my salads. Nor do I have a bag of almonds at my house to nosh on because these are densely caloric, high-protein, high-fat foods. I tell everybody I could easily be a three-hundred-pound vegan. I'm at a healthy weight because I minimize this kind of stuff in the diet.

GM: What about coconut? I'll go into a health food store and there will be all these raw desserts, these supposedly healthy alternative desserts. However, they have so much coconut in them that they'll have eighteen grams of saturated fat. Is coconut as unhealthy as it appears to be?

PP: Absolutely. It's full of saturated fat. Now, having said that, I love it. If you told me I could never have coconut again, I might have to end my life. So I don't want to give it up, but I'm very clear that it's a treat. Raw food desserts and raw food dishes in general are very high in fat. They often accomplish the textures they desire by using really high-fat foods.

This issue of food-versus-treat is something we just have to drive home. On the one hand, we certainly don't want people to think they're making a sixty-year commitment to never having dessert, birthday cake, or wedding cake, etc.; that's not going to fly. Nor do we want people stressing out thinking they blew the diet. That's a bad idea. On the other hand, this stuff can't be part of the daily fare. We need to make the whole foods our daily fare and make the treats occasional. And this is something that people get into all the time: "Well, what do you mean by occasional?" And I tell them it should be situational. Do we have a reason for having this item that is not part of the daily fare? If you graduate first in your class, a glass of champagne is okay. But today's Tuesday, it's a pretty normal day, we're not celebrating anything around here, so I think we ought to just eat our beans and rice and vegetables.

GM: On the subject of plant foods that you have to watch your intake of, what about dried fruit?

PP: There are two issues with dried fruit: First, it's high in calories. You can sit down and eat half a bag of dried apricots pretty easily. Just think about how many calories you consumed. It's like eating three dozen apricots, which you would never do. Second, you have to make sure the dried fruits you're buying aren't adulterated.

There are lots of sulfites, coloring agents, and sugar in many dried fruit products. Any time you buy cranberries that taste good right out of the package, you know that they've had sugar added to them because cranberries are actually sour. Be careful when you buy dried fruits; you don't want to be eating a lot of that stuff. Again, I'll eat it when it's in a dish. Del makes a great salad here that has raisins in it, or I'll put raisins on my oatmeal every so often. But I'm not eating handfuls of dried bananas, dried apples, dried pineapples, that kind of stuff.

GM: How about fruit juice?

PP: Never.

GM: Okay, what's wrong with fruit juice?

PP: It's concentrated calories and sugar. Instead of drinking apple juice, eat apples; instead of orange juice, eat oranges.

GM: What about salt?

PP: Well, now we get into a contentious issue. Salt restriction is one of those things that became part of the conventional wisdom; we've been told it's necessary for people to restrict salt in order to have normal blood pressure.

Early in my career, I heard Dr. McDougall buck the establishment by saying that salt restriction is not only inadvisable but may be detrimental. I got curious about it, so I reviewed the studies that had shown that salt restriction was beneficial; the difficulty was that salt restriction is usually accompanied with other dietary changes. The famous DASH (Dietary Approaches to Stop Hypertension) diet, promoted by the USDA to lower hypertension, is probably the best example of this. The participants of the

DASH study were eating more fruits and vegetables, less animal foods, higher fiber, and less salt.[50] I don't think we can attribute the improvement in their health to the salt restriction alone, when people were making so many other changes to their diet at the same time. I just really could not find a lot of clear evidence that salt restriction was important. On the other hand, according to the 2007 National Health and Nutrition Examination Survey, which included almost one hundred million adults, people who eat more salt have a lower risk of death from heart attack and stroke.[51] There are many populations on the planet that eat a lot more salt than we do that enjoy great cardiovascular health.

GM: Is Japan one of those?

PP: Japan is one of those, yes. And parts of China.

We've used salt to cure and flavor food for centuries. I don't think we can attribute our current epidemic of hypertension to salt. The bottom line is this: when you adopt the diet that we recommend, your consumption of salt is going to ratchet down quite a bit because you're not going to be eating processed meats and as much packaged foods as you were before. And another very important thing is going to happen, too—your consumption of other minerals and nutrients like potassium will go up. I think that one of the issues is the ratio of salt to other nutrients, particularly potassium, in the diet, so you're going to experience salt reduction. Also, if you salt your food at the table instead of in the cooking process, you're going to use less salt, and I think that's a good idea. In any given year, we end up with half a dozen people here who have to restrict because they really have some salt sensitivity; their blood pressure goes up when they eat salt, and it goes down when they don't.

GM: So you're not denying that that relationship could exist?

83

PP: Oh, it does exist. But as public policy, what we're doing is restricting millions of people to try to help a handful who need the restriction.

GM: Aren't we salt-restricting millions of people primarily because of their blood pressure?

PP: Well, yes, but they don't need to be restricted.[52] In other words, if they lost weight and they ate a plant-based diet without salt restriction, their blood pressure would come down naturally, without restricting it overtly. If you look at the mechanism of action for high blood pressure, a lot of it is related to damage to the endothelial tissue. If the endothelial cells can't produce nitric oxide, which is a vasodilator, the vessels start to close a little bit. Add in a little arterial plaque and the lumen in the vessels start to narrow even more; essentially, you're trying to force more blood through narrower arteries. That's the recipe for high blood pressure. Well, when you put people on a low-fat, plant-based diet, the plaque deposits stop forming and the narrowing of the lumen of the blood vessels isn't happening anymore. We stop assaulting the endothelial tissue and it starts to regenerate; it begins to produce nitric oxide and opens up those blood vessels. It's amazing, over a period of time, how many people will have their blood pressure return to normal. Add in some exercise and take off a few pounds and most people will be able to get their blood pressure down without salt restriction.

I want to mention one thing. This is not my idea—it's a Dr. McDougall idea that's worth sharing, and there's a considerable amount of evidence in the medical journals to support it.[53] Remember that our object is to encourage people to eat starchy foods and vegetables. And if salting the broccoli makes them eat a lot of it then, by gosh, let's put some salt on it. I don't want the vast majority of people who aren't salt sensitive to think they're cheating because they put salt on their broccoli and rice.

GM: What about the meat analogs: the tofu hot dogs and the Gardein meats and so forth?

PP: Well, some of them are pretty clean. Using tempeh to give spaghetti sauce the texture of something with ground meat in it, if it's a clean tempeh product, like the ones we make at Wellness Forum Foods, I don't have any problem with that. I do it; we do it here. What I have a problem with is these highly processed meat analogs that are just garbage food, like the tofu hot dogs and the fake pepperoni. Once in a while, it's not a problem. People invite me, say, to a Memorial Day picnic and they say, "Pam, we've got veggie burgers for you." They may be overly processed veggie burgers, but it's Memorial Day and people are being nice. I'm not going to die from eating a veggie burger that isn't clean. It's only when this kind of garbage infiltrates the daily diet that you don't really end up with the health improvement that you're looking for. These fake meats are transitional foods and treats. If you've got to feed your kids some tofu hot dogs to get them through the transitional period, that's fine. However, if you're still doing it two years later, you're just postponing making some serious health improvements.

GM: How do you feel about the raw food diet?

PP: That's a complicated question. What typically happens to people who adopt a raw food diet is that they do really well for a while because of all of the things that they eliminate. Many people who start a raw food diet come from eating some version of a terrible diet, so they feel really great. But then, even with the meat and the dairy out of their diet, they start to feel badly. The biggest reason they feel badly is that they can't get enough calories from eating only raw foods, or they have difficulty doing so. When they begin to feel the impact of the calorie deficiency, they start to increase their calorie count by eating nuts and oils and things of that nature. Then they start to get sick.

There are some people who are able to maintain a raw food diet well. Not everybody gets it wrong, but most people don't do it well and end up worse off as a result. I think the bigger issue is that we really don't have any evidence that shows that a raw food diet is better than a diet that includes cooked food. One of my philosophical issues around raw food is that what we're asking people to do is a big enough change all by itself, without adding layers of difficulty to it that are unnecessary. Often I find that these added layers of difficulty attract a lot of attention at the expense of things that are much more important. I think it's much more important to deal with fat in the diet, for example, than to eat all raw food. It requires an involved discussion about the effort that it takes to do the raw diet right and to teach people how to dehydrate foods and all that sort of thing; I don't see that it's worth it.

GM: I look at it this way: there are two important goals in nutrition. One is to obtain nutrients and the other is to avoid poisons or deleterious substances. Now, if you eat a lot of raw greens, vegetables, and salads, you get a lot of nutrients, which is a positive. You want to have a healthy complement of raw foods in your diet. Then if we add to these some rice, potato, or other plant food that requires cooking, there's no downside. We're not getting any poisons. We're not getting something that's high in fat or full of toxins or has animal protein or anything else. I just can't see the case for abstaining from healthy, cooked foods that satisfy our appetites, as long as we're getting our full complement of nutrient-dense raw foods.

PP: I agree with that. We want people to eat lots of salads and raw foods. But the extreme idea that you try to live on only raw foods doesn't play out really well in real life. We need those cooked foods, those cooked starchy foods, because otherwise it's difficult for the diet to be calorically adequate.

One fun dining adventure that I enjoy in many cities is to sample raw food restaurants. There are many in Los Angeles, and I've had the pleasure of dining in some of them. The food is just phenomenal at some of these places but—and this is a big but that could lead to a big butt—it's also very high in fat. If I ate at those restaurants every day, I'd be a three-hundred-pound vegan.

The whole idea of adopting a health-promoting diet is not to separate yourself from the rest of humanity and make it impossible to interact with the rest of the world. That's a terrible outcome, in my opinion. The emphasis on eating only raw food, and food combining, and a lot of other ideas that are circulating, make it harder and harder for a person to be out among the rest of the world. I don't want to stop going to family gatherings and book club, or any of the other things that I do that involve interactions and meals with other people. I don't want to adopt some eating style that's incompatible with the way the rest of the world lives. I can eat the plant-based diet we've discussed here; I can practice dietary excellence anywhere I go. I can't practice raw food-ism and food combining and a lot of these other extreme things every place I go.

GM: How do you feel about the macrobiotic diet?

PP: Well, that's interesting. There's some evidence that the macrobiotic diet is helpful for resolving cancer. We don't really have a lot of studies that point in that direction, but we have a lot of stories, enough that I think if somebody wanted to do a study on macrobiotic diets and cancer, it could be justified from a funding standpoint. It'll never happen because the drug companies will never let it happen, but I've read enough about it to believe there's something to it.

One thing that's misunderstood is that the macrobiotic diet isn't just a diet; it's a lifestyle, too. The people who have succeeded with it have not only adhered to the dietary principles but they've done a lot of the other things that are recommended in terms of the way they live their lives. I think if you're going to do macrobiotics, you're going to have to incorporate the whole program to get the benefit.

The macrobiotic diet can be difficult in terms of food preparation; it takes a lot of time. What we don't know is if it's the specific combination of foods that are included that's causing the positive effect, or if it's simply the elimination of some of the bad foods that's causing the positive effect. In other words, do we really have to do all of this, or can we get the same results from just eating a plant-based diet? I'd love to see a study with leukemia patients comparing a macrobiotic diet to our Wellness Forum plan to see if there truly is a difference between the two. Will that ever happen? No, not in this country.

GM: I lived in Boston in 1983 in a vegetarian group house near one of Michio Kushi's macrobiotic schools (Kushi founded the Kushi Institute). Whenever we advertised for a new roommate, a lot of his students would come and interview with us to see if they wanted to live in our house. They would always ask the same question: "Do you eat vegetables that grow at night?" I would say, "I don't know. I never get up to watch."

Is there anything to this "nightshade vegetable" thing? Apparently potatoes and eggplants and I'm not sure what else grow at night; is there any basis for concern about that?

PP: No, not generally. There are some patients with arthritis—it's a very small minority—who seem to do better without nightshade vegetables. I think you bring up a great example of what I was just talking about. That's a layer of difficulty added to eating a macrobiotic diet, and we just don't have any research to show that added level of restriction and difficulty is necessary most of the time. I'd love to see it studied someday; maybe I will live long enough to see the right types of studies done about diet in this country, but right now we just don't have the evidence for it.

GM: Speaking of potatoes, what's the best way to prepare a potato? Baked potato, boiled potato? Do you eat the skin, do you not eat the skin?

PP: I always eat the skin. I love potato skins. Boiled, baked, steamed—those are the ways I usually have them. But it's not necessary to eat the skin if you don't want to.

GM: Now what about a glass of wine in the evening? Anything wrong with that?

PP: Every evening is a big deal. Alcohol is not beneficial for health. The several studies that have shown that occasional drinkers are healthier than abstainers have not, I think, accounted for the fact that many abstainers are abstainers because of health conditions. I don't see a benefit from drinking, but I don't want to take the enjoyment out of life. I know some real purists, and they're a pain in the butt to be around. I don't want to be one of them. It doesn't attract people to our way of life. I enjoy an occasional cocktail and I don't discourage our members from doing so unless they have a condition like pancreatitis or hepatitis C. I think the average person can certainly drink some alcohol, but not every day.

GM: What do you say to those who believe that a daily glass of red wine explains the so-called French Paradox? They manage to eat a fatty, animal-based diet with less heart disease than Americans.

PP: First of all, the incidence of heart disease and cancer in France is very high.[54] It's lower than the United States, but it's still very high. I wouldn't be attracted to that type of risk profile. Second, the French, as well as other populations in Europe that eat similar diets, eat an enormous amount of legumes, fresh vegetables, whole grains, and fruit. The people who truly abide by this diet are not overweight. And while they eat plenty of animal foods, they eat much smaller portions than we do in America. I've spent a lot of time in Europe; I've eaten the Mediterranean diet in Europe, so I know what I'm speaking about.

Having said that, their disease rates are still high. To the extent that their health is better than ours, it's not because of the red wine or olive oil; it's because of the entire way they live their life, which includes more walking and more physical activity. It's their pattern of diet and lifestyle that is somewhat protective, not red wine and olive oil, and in any case they're not as healthy as is sometimes reported. What happens here is that people look at various diets and they read about the Mediterranean diet and say, "I like the red wine and olive oil," and they extract that and add that to the American diet, only to make things worse.

GM: Chocolate has been in the news lately because of studies that allegedly show that it's very good for the heart. That seems to be too good to be true.

PP: And it is. The danger would be people thinking they can continue to eat the fatty Western diet and then protect them-selves with fatty chocolate bars. The study that was in the news recently was a meta-analysis of seven studies. Only five of the seven showed some benefit. Even the researchers issued a caution about how to interpret the results because chocolate is high in fat and calories; even *they* did not interpret their own study as a mandate to begin eating chocolate as a preventive tool.[55] If there's some legitimate good news here, it's that if you're in good health and practicing a low-fat, plant-based diet, you can treat yourself occasionally to some chocolate without worry.

GM: What about coffee?

PP: Coffee has been a little vilified. There's no question that caffeine is a drug. As with alcohol, if you abuse it, you're going to have problems. I used to be a caffeine abuser, so I can speak to that from extreme personal experience. It used to take three pots of coffee a day to keep me going. I don't think the occasional cup of coffee is a dealbreaker. When people who are completely compliant with the diet say that a cup of coffee in the morning is something they want to do, I'm not going to make an issue out of it. To do so would be choosing the wrong battle. But when I see people drinking coffee all day long to stay awake and masking symptoms of fatigue, which should signal to them that they're overworking themselves and that their body is exhausted, I'll make an issue of that.

GM: I'm pleased to say that I've had only one cup of coffee in my life.

PP: How'd you manage that?

GM: Well, I was a seventeen-year-old high school student and visited the college I would ultimately attend, New College in Sarasota, Florida. Somebody told me that there would be a coffee klatch in the evening at the home of Professor Peggy Bates, so I went there to meet the students and some professors. Dr. Bates said to me, in front of everyone, "Glen, do you drink coffee?" Well, I never drank coffee growing up; it had never occurred to me to try it. But now I was going to college, joining the grown-ups, and I didn't want to make a fool of myself, so I had to think on my feet.

I said, "I don't know."

She said, "Well, Glen, would you like to try a cup?"

I said, "Sure."

So she gave me my first cup of coffee. And I drank a few sips. It tasted like mud. It was the worst tasting drink I'd ever experienced. I couldn't imagine that people actually drank this crap. So I never had coffee again.

Cut to twenty years later. My old literature professor was retiring, and I flew back to Sarasota to speak at his retirement dinner. I'm hanging around the campus and I meet a young woman from China who is a new student at the college. She tells me she's studying international relations with Dr. Bates. I say, "Oh, is she still here? How's she doing?"

She says, "Great. She's just the greatest professor. But she makes the worst friggin' coffee."

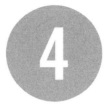

SUCCESS STORIES

· ·

GM: Pam, let's discuss how the dietary program that you recommend has worked in practice, with specific individuals. I know that, in the view of science, every individual is just an anecdote, but after a while the anecdotes begin to add up.

PP: Okay, let's start with a young lady by the name of Darcy (her name has been changed), who came to us after her condition caused her to drop out of college. She had started her menstrual period at about the average time for American girls, sometime around eleven or twelve, but from the very beginning this was just a torturous experience for her. Her periods were irregular and heavy, sometimes bleeding three weeks out of four. Then she developed severe acne and the beginnings of polycystic ovary syndrome, which is a horrific condition for a teenager to have. She graduated from high school and went off to college, but the condition worsened so much that she had to drop out of college and come back home.

Her parents found The Wellness Forum. They called and said their daughter was nineteen years old and effectively can't do anything—can't leave the house, go to school, get a job. This is quite a young age to essentially have your life be pretty much over with, so we started teaching her the diet. We cut the dairy out and got her on a low-fat, plant-based nutritional program. Within six weeks, her menstrual periods started to become regular, the horrible bleeding and the cramping started to go away, her skin cleared up, and she returned to school. She's back in nursing school now and has had a complete and total recovery. She takes no medication. So, just diet—complete and total recovery using our diet.

GM: Did she experience any other changes? Did she lose weight?

PP: Yes. She lost fifteen or twenty pounds. It's hard to know if her original weight gain had been caused by the fact that her life had come to a halt and she couldn't do anything, but now she runs, she exercises, and her skin's cleared up. She's a normal college student.

GM: Now, do you suspect that dairy had been the main culprit, or do you think it was just somehow the overall diet, all the fat and everything in the standard American diet?

PP: I think it's both. First of all, dairy foods are the worst for women with menstrual problems because dairy products by their very nature contain estrogen. Most women who have problems with hormones ranging from irregular periods to infertility are having those problems because their estrogen levels are too high. Taking in more estrogen metabolites in a glass of milk or a slice of cheese just makes the problem worse. In the case of this young lady, her entire dietary pattern was horrific. She lived on the typical college kid fare and, before that, the typical high school kid fare. The whole family, by the way, was in a similar condition. Her mother has also had a miraculous health recovery. After seeing what happened with her daughter, the mother adopted the diet and her health has turned around also. The whole family now eats this way. So a whole family of sick people became a whole family of active people eating a health-promoting diet all because their daughter had reached a crisis point.

GM: And was Darcy resistant at all, or did she immediately take to the diet?

PP: She was so anxious to have this behind her that if we had told her to graze on grass in the side yard of her house, she would have gone and done it. When people are really sick, they're really compliant because they want to heal. Somehow we've got to reach people who aren't so sick and get them to take it just as seriously. If you can make them see their choice, they'd much rather be well than become sick and have to recover.

DARCY IN HER OWN WORDS

My story started at age eleven when I started my period. By the time I was thirteen years old, I started having severe pain. I thought it was normal, but then it kept getting worse and worse every month. I began to have cramps before, during, and after my period. Some months my menstrual period would last for two-and-a-half weeks.

(cont'd. on next page)

95

(cont'd. from previous page)

I went to a gynecologist, and he gave me pain medicine, but it did not help very much. I had a laparoscopy, during which the surgeon found a cyst in my left tube and the beginning stages of endometriosis. The doctors gave me birth control pills, but I decided to stop taking them after two years because I was concerned about the health risks. All of my symptoms returned.

I began seeing a holistic health specialist, who prescribed compounded progesterone. It seemed to help for about six months, and then the symptoms returned. I tried lots of different holistic health alternatives, because I refused to go back to the doctors who never seemed to have a clear answer and always wanted to treat my symptoms instead of the actual cause. But the holistic professionals just ran tests and gave me pills and creams. Sometimes they worked for a period of time, but I usually ended up worse than when I started.

As if all of this was not bad enough, I started breaking out with acne all over my body. My face was pure red. I felt awful and tired, and at this point, the only time I got out of bed was to eat and visit doctors. I was sleeping about fourteen hours per day. I gained twenty pounds and even when I tried eating only lettuce, I could not lose the weight. My mood swings became more severe, my temper was out of control, and I began to develop sugar and thyroid problems. It seemed like I was very young to have all of these health issues.

Forced to go back to medical doctors, I was diagnosed with polycystic ovary syndrome; I had cysts all over my ovaries. This time the doctors put me back on birth control and added an antidepressant and metformin for the sugar problem.

I was absolutely desperate at this point and I continued to pray and pray, until one day a miracle came. A wonderful lady shared with me her personal recovery story with Dr. Pam Popper and The Wellness Forum. I decided to get in touch with Dr. Popper and see what might happen. By this point, I was about seven years into my journey and I would have probably tried anything. Amazingly, with Dr. Popper's diet and the exercise she asked me to do, in just six weeks my period returned—the first one in six months! I think I had the biggest smile on my face that I had had in the past three years. I was so thankful and joyful and I felt so much better. I truly felt relieved. My body was starting to work and fix itself, and, little by little, things started adjusting.

I have been on this diet for about two years and I am almost fully recovered from everything. Most of my pimples are gone, I lost the twenty pounds I had gained, and I have a lot more energy. I am able to function like a normal person. I will continue to stick to this diet for the rest of my life and I am so grateful for the transformation it has caused in my health. When things were the worst, I never thought I'd have a regular menstrual cycle or be able to get out of bed again. It is an amazing feeling to have my health restored.

GM: Now, most people come to The Wellness Forum only when they're sick.

PP: Yes. Maureen Yatwa actually came to me through my work with Rip Esselstyn and Whole Foods Market. She showed up at one of the Immersion programs last fall.

GM: That's the program that Whole Foods funds for employees with weight problems or health challenges, right?

PP: Right. Maureen, from Jacksonville, Florida, is in her forties and she had Crohn's disease—that's past tense. She qualified for the program because she also had high cholesterol and was overweight.

At the first night of Immersion, during the introductions, she stood up and said, "I'm overweight, I have high cholesterol, and I also have Crohn's disease. My daughter, who's a teenager, also has Crohn's disease, and I want both of us to get better." So I went up to her after the opening-night dinner, introduced myself, and said, "In order to fix the Crohn's disease, you'll have to accept a little bit more dietary restriction than the others because gluten is contraindicative for Crohn's. So the oats and some of the other things we have here, you're not going to be able to eat. But there's plenty of food here; you're not going to starve. There are just some things you can't have." Everybody at the Immersion is on a whole food, low-fat, plant-based diet, but she would have just a little bit more restriction.

There are all kinds of activities planned at the Immersion, canoeing and field trips and so forth. Maureen didn't sign up for any of it because if you're a Crohn's patient, your disease is not under control. You can't go anywhere because you have to be by the bathroom. It's a debilitating disease. The forty-five-minute bus ride into town—you can't do that. You can't be out on a canoe. Life revolves around locating the nearest bathroom.

By the time the midweek came, she was well enough to do those things. She showed significant improvement within in a matter of days. Today, she not only doesn't have Crohn's disease but she doesn't take medication for it, she's lost the weight, and her cholesterol is down. And her daughter, who was on her way to duplicating mom at the age of seventeen or eighteen, also no longer has Crohn's disease.

GM: So in just a few days the Crohn's was gone? Crohn's often stays with people for how long?

PP: Their whole lives. The trajectory of Crohn's and ulcerative colitis and these inflammatory bowel diseases is discouraging. There may be periods of some remission, where it gets a little bit better, but it always progresses, and the drugs get stronger. It's not unusual to use Remicade infusions, which are immunosuppressants, very strong drugs. And when that fails, they start taking portions of the bowel out; they remove the inflamed portion. And obviously, there's an end point to that; there's only so much you can take out before you don't have a GI tract or intestines anymore. That's where Maureen was headed, and her situation was obviously pretty acute. If you're afraid of a forty-five-minute bus ride because you're not going to be near a bathroom, you're pretty far down the road. So she totally recovered. She talks about it very openly, as she should since she can be a real inspiration to others who have this condition.

MAUREEN YATWA IN HER OWN WORDS

I met Dr. Pam Popper while participating in a program sponsored by my employer. There were several reasons why I wanted to participate in this program, and one of them was that I had Crohn's disease for nineteen years. During that time I was medicated with steroids, antibiotics, and other

(cont'd. on next page)

(cont'd. from previous page)

medications; would have flare-ups; and was even hospitalized a few times. In 1993 I had my gallbladder removed. My Crohn's had advanced so much that I was hospitalized with toxic shock syndrome and had twelve inches of my intestines removed in an emergency surgery. The infection was so severe that the wound was left open to heal; I was left with a horrible scar. From that point, I routinely had visited the bathroom between six and fourteen times per day, and my stomach was always sore and bloated; I just accepted that this was my fate. I had to always be near a restroom. The anxiety I experienced would cause me to shake, sweat, and feel guilty because I was always making my family wait while I found a bathroom. A class trip with my children was a heinous experience.

Dr. Pam told me the very first time we met that I could get better and that she would help me figure out what to eat and what not to eat. The program I attended lasted for five days; by the end of this time, my Crohn's disease was better. I maintained a plant-strong diet after the program and my Crohn's disease completely went away!

For the first time in nineteen years, I am not running for the bathroom and I have the freedom to do anything I want to do. I can watch my daughter's whole soccer game without running to a restroom. This has totally changed my life.

Getting rid of the Crohn's disease is not the only positive change: I've lost nineteen pounds and my blood pressure and cholesterol dropped to ideal levels.

I wish I'd known about this earlier, but I'm grateful to have my life back.

GM: I take it that The Wellness Forum attracts a lot of people with digestive or bowel disorders?

PP: We do. Jill Collett is a yoga teacher at our studio who had ulcerative colitis. She'd been on and off medication for it. Her ulcerative colitis had progressed to the place where the inflammation in the bowel started to affect other parts of the body; she developed some inflammation in her eyes and her vision became a bit impaired, something that can't be fixed. Jill had been a student at our yoga studio for a long time, but I didn't know, until she started our yoga-training program and spoke with me about it, that she had been suffering for twenty years with ulcerative colitis.

Jill didn't eat a terrible diet, but it wasn't perfect. Remember the combination lock theory; you know, you've got to get all four numbers right. You can't do 75 percent. We helped her make that additional 25 percent of dietary improvement; it took only three weeks for her stools to become solid and for her to stop suffering from ulcerative colitis—off the meds and everything's fine. And she's been fine ever since. She actually made the comment that her energy level was so high that she was starting to scare her husband. This had been a twenty-year problem for her; after only twenty-one days on the diet, she was in great shape. You could really see the difference, too. Her face, her complexion changed a lot after this period of time; now she just looks phenomenally great.

JILL COLLETT IN HER OWN WORDS

When I talked with Pam Popper regarding my gut issues for the first time, I thought I was faring well with my ulcerative

(cont'd. on next page)

(cont'd. from previous page)

colitis. I thought I felt as good as possible given my condition. For nearly twenty years, I had accepted stomach cramps, bloating, and occasional sprints to the toilet as part of who I was. I learned to breathe through cramps, dress for the bloat, and I could tell you where the nearest restroom was in any public venue, including the Roman Colosseum (across the street in the train station). I also accepted the fact that once every few years, I would wake up in the morning and a bit more of my eyesight would be gone. All these symptoms were due to the disease diagnosed in my twenties as ulcerative proctitis and then the progression to ulcerative colitis as the years passed.

When I first mentioned something to Pam about my condition, I was taking a maintenance medication that I had been on for several years following my last vision loss. I took it to stave off any systemic inflammation and to preserve my remaining eyesight. I had been through all sorts of drugs beginning in my twenties with the sulfas, using suppositories for flares and muscle relaxants for cramps. I had had colonoscopies, MRIs, spinal taps, tons of blood work, flown to see top doctors, all with the same outcome: use the maintenance drugs, try to minimize stress and known triggers, and hope for the best. I ate fairly well, didn't drink caffeine, had the occasional glass of wine, and exercised regularly. So why did I still wake with cramps, deal with the "food baby," and have irregular BMs?

Through Pam and The Wellness Forum, I learned that I could soothe and even cure my inflamed system with just a few changes. She said, "You can get rid of this." Those were the game-changing words; well, those and, "You can never let dairy or gluten pass your lips again." I had minimized my direct dairy intake in the past, but never had I been told so bluntly that what I ate had such a profound effect. It wasn't just minimize or try to avoid—it was an absolute. No gluten, no hidden dairy, nothing baked in, melted, sprinkled, etc. It makes perfect sense now. Stop annoying the intestines and they will stop annoying me. While I had always eaten what I thought was a "healthy" diet, I cleaned it up even further to become more plant-centered.

Since that first meeting, I have been careful to stick with the absolutes, and my system is functioning amazingly well. No more cramps, no more runs to the nearest bathroom, and, best of all, my energy level is through the roof. I find it easy to stick with the plan since I feel so much better as a result. I do not miss greasy cheese, ice cream, or the aftermath of indulging. Not worth it at all. Feeling good is an amazing motivator.

GM: So these have been examples of people who look better and feel better and get their lives back. Another bragging point you make for the diet is clarity of mind . . .

PP: Okay, I've got a story on the subject. I love this story. The man's name is Barry Small, and I've been friends with his wife, Elisabeth, for twenty-two years. I met Barry because one of my best friends married him. I was at their wedding and I'm a frequent guest at their house. So over the years, their diet has changed some as a result of my influence; they never were Mc-Donald's-eating people or anything like that, but they also never ate optimally; I think they always looked at me as an extremist. They took the more moderate road to health and were able to do pretty well. They never were very sick or obese or anything. They never consulted with me much about health issues. When I was in their house, we always ate the low-fat vegan food, but I knew from what was in the freezer that they weren't really on our diet. And these people, by the way, adopted a boy and a girl from Russia. Barry became a parent again at the age of sixty, which is a keen motivation to stay healthy.

One day I got a call from Barry and Elisabeth; they're really worried. Barry's concern was that a couple of times he was on a conference call for work and his mind went blank. He said, "I completely skipped out and I couldn't even get words out of my mouth. It took a couple minutes for me to come back to the present and I'm very concerned because I felt like an idiot." It also happened once when he was talking in front of a group. He told me he had been going to the Cleveland Clinic; Barry has good insurance and boy, will these high-end hospitals use it up. He explained that he's got high cholesterol and blood pressure, so immediately it's clear this is a cardiovascular issue. He overnights me his files; they were so extensive that they had to come in a box. I sat down one night and I read through the patient files; it was test after test and image after image. They spent $10,000 to $20,000 on all this imaging and testing and it all said the same thing: he had high cholesterol and high blood pressure, he had gained weight over the years, and he had cardiovascular disease that had been progressing for decades.

I got Barry and Elisabeth on the phone and told them what I thought. I said, "What's wrong with you is very simple: you have high cholesterol and high blood pressure—it's a marker for coronary artery disease. You're having impaired oxygenation to the brain. These moments when you check out and it takes you two minutes to come back, I think it's all vascular."

We went through the low-fat vegan diet, and he listened hard because he was scared. He said, "I've got kids, I've got to get myself squared away." Fear can be a really good motivator. He said, "I promise I will do everything starting with the next morsel I put into my mouth. You'll get my complete cooperation; I'm going to do this thing." It didn't take very long. He went back to his doctor after about three months. He had lost twenty-five pounds. He said he had to go out and buy all new clothes. All of those thought and speech symptoms he was having totally disappeared. Within three months, he went back to the doctor at the Cleveland Clinic and went off all his blood pressure and cholesterol-lowering meds. His cholesterol dropped like a rock and his blood pressure was healthfully low to normal. The doctor did the brachial artery tourniquet test on him and told Barry, "I think there's a mistake. Last time you were in here you had advancing coronary artery disease and now, my God, it's like you have the arteries of an eighteen-year-old." And so they did the test again and it was exactly the same result. Barry completely reversed his coronary artery disease.

And he tells me that every time people see him now, they say, "Oh my God, what did you do? What happened to you? You look fabulous!" And Elisabeth was never really overweight, but because the family converted to the diet, she's also dropped a few pounds. They look like a Hollywood couple now. They're just in phenomenal shape and, of course, they've got kids in high school and want to stay young and healthy and see their kids graduate from high school and college and get married and all of that good stuff. In fact, they're thinking of adopting some more children now because they're feeling so great. And his cholesterol is so low that he gets the usual response from the people in the medical field, "Oh my gosh, Barry, that cholesterol is so low it's probably dangerous." He laughs. He read Rip Esselstyn's book and he trusts me. So he laughs. He says, "Yeah, yeah, four months

105

ago my cholesterol was high like you think it ought to be. I was a candidate for bypass surgery. Now you're telling me you want me to go back there?"

GM: He sounds like a good case of someone who's seen too many doctors.

PP: Yeah. While I don't discourage people from seeing doctors, many just need to be taught the diet. What Barry needed was not more doctors; he needed to get the salmon and the olive oil out of the house and to stop fooling himself. He just needed to stop all that stuff; it's amazing how fast people get better if they do. One of the reasons why that's a favorite story is because everybody in our field wants to help the people close to them, but it can be very frustrating when people who are complete strangers listen to you and heal, while the people who are closest to you are harder to reach. You'd like to say something, but you don't want to lecture them every time you see them. I love these people. I've known Elisabeth for twenty-something years and I've known Barry for half that time; it would be devastating to me if something happened to either of them. So, you know, these are close, close friends. Now he's better, and that makes me very happy. But sometimes you have to wait until the time is right.

BARRY SMALL IN HIS OWN WORDS

I am sixty-three years old. I have had high cholesterol, hypertension, and weight problems for several years and they had been getting worse. In August 2010, my total cholesterol was 264, my LDL was 186, and my triglycerides were 147. I was being medicated for these conditions, but my health was continuing to deteriorate.

In September 2010, I was told that I was getting close to needing bypass surgery. This was not something I was willing to do; I have a great wife and two great kids who need their dad. My health risks had to be addressed, so I decided to look into other options.

My wife, Elisabeth, and I have known Dr. Pam Popper for many years; Pam's a close family friend. She had influenced our eating habits over the years. We talked often about how powerful diet could be in preventing and treating disease. But we had never really made the great leap to being vegan or near-vegan. Now, though, faced with the prospect of worsening health and a surgery I did not want to have, I decided to talk to her about my health.

I sent her my blood tests and other medical information and on December 2, 2010, she called me to give her recommendations. I'll never forget what Pam said to me: "Are you ready to do what it takes to get better?" I respected her opinion, so when she said, "Never let another bite of animal food, processed food, or oil pass your lips again," that was when I immediately became an oil-free vegan.

Only ninety days later, I went to my family physician to get a lipid profile blood test. A few days later, he called me to come in and review the results. In his office, the first thing he said was, "Hippocrates was right! Food is your medicine." My cholesterol went from 197 (on medication) to 157. He also did an arterial elasticity test, and it showed that I once again had flexible arteries. He said it was completely different from my test a few months earlier.

(cont'd. on next page)

(cont'd. from previous page)

The weight loss was also impressive. After ninety days, I had trimmed down from a size 38-inch waist to a 33-inch waist. I am now the weight I was in college forty-five years ago. I now take no medications, and people constantly tell me I look twenty years younger than I used to.

It was amazing to me that a problem that I had been dealing with for twenty years vanished in only ninety days on a plant-based diet.

PP: I met Patty Yeager in Las Vegas a few years ago; when we first met, she was very overweight. After my visit, she became a Wellness Forum member and learned our eating plan. I was in Las Vegas the following year for a *Forks Over Knives* screening, and Patty was there. She had lost so much weight and changed so much I walked right by her and did not recognize her. Patty was always attractive, even when she was overweight, but when she lost the weight, she became drop-dead gorgeous.

PATTY YEAGER IN HER OWN WORDS

I took the Wellness 101 class about a year and a half ago, and my eating habits started changing as soon as I started taking the classes. One of the first things I did was to get rid of all processed foods in my pantry. I had already stopped eating most meat, but after only two weeks, I decided to eliminate fish, too. The last thing I gave up was dairy. I was a frozen yogurt addict, but was really surprised when I decided to treat myself to it a few months after giving it up—it tasted awful! It was the same for so many things that were a part of my regular diet, like soda pop, cheese, yogurt, and other foods. I had heard over and over that your taste buds change, but I really didn't believe it until it happened to me. I am now so attuned to my body that when I have that occasional treat, like a candy bar, I can immediately feel my body turning into a sugar-craving machine for the next few days. In fact, I used to feel that way ALL the time and I'm so glad I no longer live feeling that way! Usually after the sugar craving, a feeling of sluggishness would follow, and I found myself not wanting to do much of anything. I am SO happy not to be in that cycle anymore!

Probably the most surprising thing I learned in the Wellness 101 class was that I could eat a significantly larger quantity of the right foods and still lose weight. By learning the RIGHT things to eat, you never really overindulge and you feel satisfied. In fact, I feel like I eat all the time and I've never looked better or felt healthier.

I was fortunate that I did not have any pending "medical health problems" and that I was doing this for prevention purposes for my kids and for myself, but I was concerned about extra weight I had put on. I definitely have lost weight, I am never tired, and I feel good all the time. It is interesting that when you feel this way, you notice even more how many people around you are always tired, complaining, have a negative attitude, and are always running to their doctor to have prescriptions filled for every little ache and pain. I KNOW that a change in nutrition would turn ALL of that around. My mind

(cont'd. on next page)

(cont'd. from previous page)

feels clearer and my body feels healthy. I am never sick and I am never ever tired. I want everyone to feel the way I do, which is why I am headed down the path to share this lifestyle with as many people as I can! I feel very blessed to have learned this information before I was in the sick care system and I feel doubly blessed that my children will live their whole lives with these healthy habits!

When I was asked what is my favorite dish or food, I can definitely say it's a tie between my morning smoothies and a big brown rice bowl, both of which are amazing and SO filling! Did I mention—I'm never hungry!

Being a single mom with four children, I do make an effort to get at least seven hours of sleep and I work out at least five to six times a week. I hike, bike, run (well more like a slow jog, but at least I try), attend yoga classes, and lift weights. The better you start to feel, the MORE you want to do physical activity and you actually see and feel the difference in your mind and body when you don't get the workout in.

When asked how my family and friends have responded to my new habits, I can honestly say, "Some have and some have not." Sometimes, as we know, the people who need the help the most are the most resistant. I have learned that strong-arming someone into this lifestyle, if they are not ready to hear the information, will never work. I have chosen instead to live by example. I think people who meet me and feel the energy and happiness that I exude—largely because of this plant-strong lifestyle—will get people who want a change to ask for the help and get educated and make the change. I know for sure that if I CAN DO IT, anyone can!

Finally, when I was asked what advice do I have for other people who are considering becoming Wellness Forum members, I can say without hesitation there is nothing to lose. Get the education, then decide, make small changes, make big changes, DO something. If you continue to do what you have always done you will continue to get the same results. Why not try something that WORKS?

I am very fortunate to have come in contact with The Wellness Forum and Dr. Popper. Everyone should take advantage of the opportunity and make a life-altering decision to not only "look" healthy but BE healthy!

PP: Martin (his name has been changed) is a restaurant manager in his fifties who lives in California. He has hepatitis C and was advised to undertake interferon therapy because his viral load was very, very high and escalating. His liver enzymes were up. If you look at the track record for interferon therapy for hepatitis C, it's effective about 40 percent of the time, and the side effects are horrible. So you've got a 60 percent failure rate and you're stuck with the side effects. Martin decided that he didn't want to do it and called me.

We put him on a low-fat vegan diet, to which he has been faithfully compliant. Martin's really good about it. Long story short, even his traditional docs leave him alone now because nothing's changed; his disease hasn't progressed at all. This is an instructive story not only because the diet worked so well but also because it reminds you that the disease can kill you only if it progresses. Even if your enzymes are still elevated and your viral load is a little high, it's not going anywhere; you'll probably live to ninety-five and die of something else. Martin will not die from liver failure.

GM: I didn't know that hepatitis C isn't as much of a threat if you're on this diet because—

PP: Because it doesn't progress. A major problem in the health care business is the tendency to want to get rid of disease at almost any cost. Sometimes in the process of getting rid of it we kill the patient; this is often the case with cancer. Many times it's better to just keep the disease at bay because if it doesn't progress, it can't kill you.

GM: And that's a lesson that many are learning with prostate cancer.

PP: Yeah. I've seen a lot of people who are not cured, but they're not dying, either. Martin's a good example of that. His HCV RNA, a measure of his hepatitis viral load, actually declined between 2006 and 2011, from 6.74 to 6.21, respectively. His ALT (alanine transaminase), a liver enzyme whose increased levels mirror worsening disease, similarly declined from 87 to 75 in the same period. As aggressive as his hepatitis was, he could have been either on interferon therapy or dead by now, and he's neither of those things. The failure rate for the usual drug treatment is quite high, around 60 percent, and there are serious side effects; there are good reasons to avoid this treatment. Instead of fighting that losing battle, he's out surfing and living life—and loving it. His doctors used to nag him to try new medications, but he stuck with the program. Since it's now clear that the condition is not worsening, his doctors have learned to leave him alone.

MARTIN IN HIS OWN WORDS

I contracted hepatitis C many years ago from intravenous drug use. I have been clean for many years, but, of course, I am still concerned about this illness. My traditional doctors recommended a one-year treatment program with interferon, but I was reluctant to do this because of the side effects and the fact that the treatment is often not very effective.

I decided to look for alternatives and, shortly after, I met Dr. Pam Popper at a health conference. After listening to her speak, I was convinced that diet was a big influence on health and decided to consult with her. After doing so, I adopted the plant-based diet she recommended with a few additional suggestions to address the hepatitis C. The results have been amazing. The hepatitis C has been arrested (my viral load decreased and then has remained constant ever since), my cholesterol went from 182 to 151, and my homocysteine was lowered to 8. At the age of sixty-five, I am healthier than I was at twenty-five. I also followed Dr. Pam's advice about exercise—I do aerobic exercise, lift weights, and practice yoga for flexibility.

I'm glad I did not subject myself to drug treatment—the results from the diet are much better, and there were no risks involved.

PP: Ellen Seigel is an interesting story. There are two reasons I wanted to talk about her. The first is that, unlike most members of The Wellness Forum who join because they have health issues, Ellen really had no diseases or conditions. She did want to lose some weight, but mainly she just decided she wanted to stay healthy. Her story is also interesting because her husband, by contrast, did have some health issues and he initially chose not to adopt the diet. I think this is a situation many people face; they are ready for change, but their spouse or significant other is not, which can make life more difficult.

I met Ellen when she moved to Columbus from New York. Some mutual friends suggested that she come to my yoga studio and get to know me. She did, we became friends, and as a result, she joined The Wellness Forum. She adopted the plant-based diet, started working out with me at our gym, and continued to come to yoga.

Her husband, however, was not ready to change his eating habits or to exercise.

Over a period of about a year, Ellen's physical appearance changed a lot—she lost a lot of weight and developed that bright-eyed, energetic "I'm a plant eater" look we've all seen. Her husband continued to eat animal foods and stay on his meds.

Ellen is a therapist and has been married for forty years, so she knew better than to try to tell Gary what to do. Eventually, her patience paid off. Gary started eating more plant food, he lost weight, and his cholesterol and blood pressure went down; now the plant-based diet is one more thing they share.

ELLEN SEIGEL IN HER OWN WORDS

I had been practicing yoga off and on for a year or so. When my son went away to college, I searched for studios in Columbus so I could take a class when visiting. I discovered The Wellness Forum hot yoga; those classes are what eventually led me to meeting Dr. Popper.

My previous health/fitness background can be summed up in one word: inconsistency. I had been a vegetarian on and off for years and I never exercised regularly. I joined The Wellness Forum and took the Wellness 101 class with the tender attitude of, "I'll let this information wash through me and I'll see what sticks." I had schooled myself on "so-called" nutrition over the years and now was ready to take in new information. I was pleasantly surprised; I felt the new ideas were registering. I was making changes gradually. All of a sudden, the idea hit me that I couldn't go on weighing 165 pounds. Gradual was no longer enough. I retook the Wellness 101 class and started to strictly follow the program. I also began to train with Pam. I participated in yoga regularly and lost twenty to twenty-five pounds within a short time. I never in my life felt "athletic," so I was delighted and surprised when I was awarded with "yoga student of the month"!

I worked hard during yoga to see and embrace the benefits of working with my body while relaxing my mind. It's always wise to keep your spirits up and look for ways to turn challenges you've undertaken (changing to dietary excellence and exercise) into fun, enjoyment, and gratification.

While I continue to remain consistent with this dietary excellence, I still eat a little too much—it all tastes so good. I am continuing to improve both my eating and yoga practice. My family is amazed and impressed with the consistency of my eating right and exercising. The key to this, I believe, is keeping my active connection with "everything" Wellness Forum.

My husband, Gary, was not one to be a vegetarian or to exercise. Gary had three stents put in fifteen years ago and

(cont'd. on next page)

(cont'd. from previous page)

never felt the need to drastically modify his eating or his relaxed, sedentary lifestyle. At my invitation, he agreed to take the Wellness 101 class with me. I was happily surprised that he agreed. He also heard Pam talk at a few of the WF dinners and then, after we saw *Forks Over Knives,* I witnessed the most amazing transformation in him. He started to take brisk walks for an hour daily, significantly reduced his consumption of animal foods, lost fifteen pounds, and reduced his medications significantly. He even orders pizza without the cheese . . . and finds it satisfactory. I'm impressed!

While Gary had good reasons to change, I never thought he'd ever change. So I worked on myself. One of the things that tickles me the most is Gary saying, "I'm fixing salad. Can I cut some up for you?" I have a new closeness with my husband in an area I least expected. Sharing the food preparation and dietary excellence is amazing and wonderful.

My advice to anyone who is considering this type of change is to take yourself seriously and get moving on it—the sooner the better. A healthy and happy life awaits you. I was fortunate enough to change my ways when my only problem was being overweight—I did not have other serious diseases. And don't make your plans based on others, even those close to you. In my case, my husband was not interested at all and eventually joined me because he saw the wisdom in it for himself. Sometimes someone has to go first, and maybe that someone needs to be you.

PP: Cat Timmons has an inspiring story. This one goes back a long time; we've been following her for a while. She joined The

Wellness Forum in her early thirties when she was battling leukemia. She was receiving chemotherapy, which was making her worse. The leukemia was also getting worse; the situation had progressed to the place where she had a lot of infection in her mouth (cancer patients often get infections because of the chemotherapy). As a result of the infection of her mouth, her teeth were starting to break off at the root. She couldn't chew. She was in devastatingly poor health and went to the doctor, who told her it was worse than ever. Cat went home, got on her knees on the floor of her house, and prayed to God, "I'm going to die unless something else happens and if I'm destined to live, please send something my way because I really do want to live, God. And if you're up there, hearing me, send something."

She went to a networking meeting the next day and met somebody who works for The Wellness Forum. She came to The Wellness Forum, adopted the low-fat, plant-based diet, while continuing her chemotherapy treatments, and made remarkable progress. She had to puree all her food because her teeth were so compromised that she couldn't chew. In six weeks, the situation turned around enough that she wanted to stop the chemotherapy treatment. Her husband was concerned and her doctors were hysterical because they believed that chemotherapy was her only hope; they attributed the success she'd had to the chemo, not the diet. She got them to agree that she could stay off the drugs for a week and see what happened; she promised to go back on chemo if her condition deteriorated. But her condition continued to improve, so she never went back on the chemo.

In time, she made a complete recovery from the leukemia. She eventually had implants; now her whole mouth is fully restored. But when a woman undergoes chemotherapy, she undergoes early menopause. Cat was only in her thirties when this happened, and was clearly never going to have any children. Well, she stayed with the low-fat, plant-based diet and eventually the menopause

117

reversed itself. She now has a four-year-old. We call these kids who weren't supposed to be born Wellness Forum babies; we all feel like they're our own. Every time Cat comes into the office with this kid, he's fawned over by all our people because he really is a miracle baby. So that's Cat's story; she's just living her life now. This is all really behind her. She even testified in front of an Ohio legislative committee about allowing nondieticians to talk about nutrition. She testified the day after she had surgery for the implants and said, "I want to tell you something. Two years ago I was almost dead and yesterday I underwent all this surgery and yet today I can stand up and tell you my story. So you need to pay attention."

CAT TIMMONS IN HER OWN WORDS

Things were going well in my life. I had money, success, an expanding business, family, friends, a decent home, plus time to play and enjoy life.

Then, in 2002, I contracted a viral infection in my sinuses. My doctors began treating me for a sinus infection. I consumed several rounds of antibiotics. X-rays and CAT scans showed that the infection was spreading throughout my facial features, specifically my jawbones. The infection was causing deterioration of my jaw and teeth. A biopsy of the infected area soon revealed cancerous cells.

At this point, the doctors did not want to perform surgery to remove the infection because of the fear of exposing the cancerous cells to other parts of my body. They wanted to try to find a medicine that would eliminate the infection. But none worked. So ultimately, the infection mutated and spread throughout my body: a cancer called acute lymphatic leukemia.

This diagnosis changed the treatment plan altogether. Now my new doctors wanted to treat me with chemotherapy. Soon after, I became physically unable to keep up with my daily routine. I was tired, sick to my stomach, feverish, and mentally confused. I was told that these symptoms were normal in my condition.

I began to lose jobs because I could not keep up with the work. My medical bills began to pile up because my insurance would pay only a portion of the actual cost. My prescription co-pays rose to $3,000 each for a four- to six-week supply of medicine. And I was feeling worse instead of better. That's when the depression began to set in.

My heart was in turmoil. I was a good person, and yet my life was being dismantled and taken away. Everything I had worked so hard for was being stripped from me. My life savings, my clients, my possessions, my mental stability, my health—all gone.

A business associate introduced me to someone who worked at The Wellness Forum who became my "wellness coach" and talked to me about how important diet was in regaining my health, and that I had to work on my mind, body, and spirit if I wanted to get well. I made a personal choice to begin changing my eating habits and attempted to begin healing through nutrition and herbal therapy.

During the next several weeks, I implemented a powerful blend of natural plant foods into my diet. And I stuck to it. Every day, for every meal, I blended these foods into a smoothie. I had already been on a liquid diet for months,

(cont'd. on next page)

(cont'd. from previous page)

so this was easy for me to implement. Six weeks to the day, I woke up and I actually felt better. I began to feel new hope and excitement.

Now I had to make a decision whether to continue chemotherapy or to stop this treatment and rely completely on food, herbs, and faith. My family begged me not to stop the doctor's treatment plan because they were concerned for my health. So I made a deal with them—give me just one week. I will do what I want to do for one week. If my blood tests were worse, then I would continue with the chemotherapy. If my blood tests were the same or better, then they were to leave me alone and let me continue with alternatives. Agreed.

The doctor said, with anger, that if I were to stop treatment now, I would certainly die. Since I was so sick, so broke, and three days from losing my home, death did not seem like a bad alternative to me.

One week later, my blood tests were just slightly better. Not worse, though! I received my family's blessing to continue my own treatment plan. A couple of months later, my blood tests showed great improvements. My infection and my cancer cells were beginning to dissolve.

One year later, I was infection free and cancer free! Not only that but my allergies were going away, my arthritis was improving, and many other ailments were nonexistent.

But the story doesn't end there. When I was a teenager, I had many surgeries to eliminate cysts in my uterus and ovaries. I was left with 90 percent scar tissue. I was told that having children would be impossible. Well, with just six months of healing from my last surgery, I found out that I was pregnant. I was in shock. When I told my husband, there was silence. He then said that whatever decision I make, he would support me. I told my husband that the decision has already been made. God would not put me through all this only to let me and my unborn child die now. So, as my doctors explained the serious dangers of this pregnancy and the case for terminating it, my faith just became stronger.

As part of the high-risk pregnancy, we had an opportunity to evaluate my uterus. To our amazement, the doctors could find no scar tissue. They even had my old X-rays showing the scar tissue. Now there was none. As we began to try to explain this, we realized that some herbs I was taking had actually healed the scarring and enhanced my fertility.

At thirty-nine years of age, after eighteen years of marriage, I delivered a beautiful, healthy baby boy. My son is now four years old. Along with us, he eats all natural, organic foods, and he likes it.

I am now working part-time from home and raising my son. I always look forward to sharing with him how to be healthy and happy.

PP: Janet Triner is a schoolteacher in Chicago. I chose this story because as a teacher, she really cared about paying it forward. She had a gastrointestinal disorder—lots of diarrhea, gas, discomfort, nausea, and that sort of thing. We attract a lot of members who have GI disorders because so many have been helped after adopting our diet. Fortunately, Janet had not progressed to the point where she had had surgeries or been hospitalized, but she was plenty miserable.

And so it was just a nice clean deal. When Janet learned how to eat right, she found that she didn't have these problems anymore. But Janet teaches in this elementary school and felt that the kids should have a different view of nutrition than they have. In the past when she'd raise the subject, her colleagues would make fun of her. All the same, she began to talk about nutrition to her kids and was willing to take the flak. I told her that what often helps us in the schools is somebody with some staying power who keeps pressing for nutritional changes until he or she gets a chance to have some influence. So she got herself appointed the wellness coordinator for her school. She called me and said, "Pam, now everybody has to listen to me." She's managed to train a lot of teachers; she's teaching them about plant-based nutrition and is getting them to talk about it in the classroom. Janet has converted her own success story into one that has really influenced countless kids. They're all experiencing a different view of nutrition now because Janet got well and became passionate.

JANET TRINER IN HER OWN WORDS

I was a person who was very much caught in the medical mill that Dr. Popper talks about. I had a lot of GI problems and I had a lot of allergy problems. Doctors were always doing all kinds of tests; I would have CT scans and other tests to see what was going on in my abdomen. From about the age of twenty, I was having irritable bowel symptoms, and they just kept giving me medicine.

I heard Dr. Popper speak at a conference and I was just fascinated. Soon after that, I was diagnosed with asthma and I was put on inhalers and medicine and I was having abdominal pain. My OB/GYN thought it was endometriosis and she wanted to do surgery, and another doctor thought it was a hernia and he couldn't see it on the test but he was sure if he could get in there he could find it. I called Dr. Popper's Wellness Forum and set up an appointment and she talked to me on the phone. I thought I was eating a healthy diet, but she said, "I can see why you're so sick." I was eating tons of dairy and I was eating tons of sugar because I'm very thin and was able to eat stuff like that and not gain weight. She said, "You have to cut out sugar. You have to cut out dairy. You have to cut out gluten." She described the diet I had to eat to heal my gut, and I changed my diet that day. I stopped that night and then I started eating the healing diet and taking a probiotic.

My asthma symptoms disappeared and then my abdominal issues eventually completely disappeared. I have not had to have more tests; I have not had to go back on medicine. I have a much better body. I am healthy, I am educated, I have been able to educate my family, and we've all gotten healthier because of that.

In addition to my own health issues, I'm a teacher concerned about children. I had received training on brain function through my school district, which included only a passing mention that protein was needed for brain function. But after taking classes from The Wellness Forum, I was convinced that children needed to eat a better diet in order for their brains to function well. I decided to attend The Wellness Forum's conference on children's nutrition and at that conference I met so many people who had made a difference in their school district and I realized that I wanted to do that, too.

(cont'd. on next page)

(cont'd. from previous page)

I returned home and talked to someone in our central office who told me that we'd need to organize a committee to change school lunches. I am very shy, so I surprised myself when I said I would head that committee. During my tenure, we changed school meals, which meant changing food service providers.

Lunches definitely improved—kids were offered whole wheat products, rice, vegetables, and fruit. The food service provider even agreed to do food-tasting events for the kids.

We instituted a wellness class for kids and provided a training program for parents. I've given presentations to our teachers at teacher meetings. I, of course, use information on healthy diets in my own classroom and now teachers come to me for information on what to do in their classrooms.

I tell everyone who will listen that we are educators—we teach kids how to read, how to write, and how to do math; we should be teaching them how to make good food choices, too.

PP: Some of the work we do is in employer settings. Employers pay for employees to take our classes in order to improve their health and lower their insurance costs. For example, the city of Dublin, Ohio, a suburb of Columbus, is a client of The Wellness Forum. As with our other employer clients, we have had some incredible successes. One of those people is Larry Nicol. Larry decided to take our Wellness 101 class at work, and here's what happened to him.

LARRY NICOL IN HIS OWN WORDS

When I heard Dr. Pam Popper's talk to our employees in early 2012, I thought she was talking directly to me. My numbers were barely good enough to pass the "Healthy by Choice" criteria at work, so it was time to make a change. Although my wife and I had tried other diets without much success, we thought this was worth a try.

When I told my wife I wanted to do this, her response was, "What are we going to eat?" Meat, dairy, and oil were staples of our diet. For a while, it seemed like all we ate was beans and rice. But gradually, we learned through the classes to make substitutions and how to shop for healthier options. We increased our consumption of fruit, vegetables, whole grains, and legumes, and we decreased our intake of animal foods. We now eat meat only once or twice per week instead of every day.

We've found that plant-based recipes are easy to find and we've actually enjoyed experimenting with new meals and foods. The biggest challenge for my wife was eliminating dairy, but we've both learned to focus on what we can have, instead of what we can't. And there are plenty of good choices.

Just eight weeks into the program, I felt better than I have in a very long time and I was fitting into clothes I had not worn for twenty years. I am not taking any medications and now food is my medicine. I will never go back to my previous diet—for one thing, I'm in control of my food instead of any food controlling me. And also I feel so good now and I never want to go back to feeling bad again.

(cont'd. on next page)

(cont'd. from previous page)

Some people have told me they think the diet is drastic, but I tell them that everyone should look in the mirror and say to themselves, "No one cares as much about me as I do." If you do that, then this program is worth it, and the benefits far outweigh the efforts.

GM: Did the other participants in the Dublin program do as well?

PP: Yes, they did. The compliance rate was over 90 percent for the group. After only eight weeks, eight individuals reduced or eliminated their medications for conditions like type 2 diabetes and hypertension, and two had scheduled appointments with their docs to discuss their meds. All of the overweight participants lost weight, and one person lost more than twenty-seven pounds. The city scheduled more classes for employees who became interested after seeing their peers get such incredible results. Just think if every employer in America offered this program—we could make employer-sponsored health care plans affordable really quickly!

GM: What's your best weight-loss story?

PP: That would be Del, our Chef Del Sroufe. Del's story is still unfolding.

GM: I saw him on YouTube.

PP: Well, now he's even thinner. He's down to 250 from 475.

GM: In how much time?

PP: In five years.

GM: How tall is he?

PP: About six-three. So at 210 or 215, he'll be gorgeous. There are so many aspects of Del's story that are interesting. Let's start with the fact that he was a 475-pound vegan, living proof that you can be vegan and still be profoundly unhealthy. Being vegan doesn't mean anything if you don't do it right. Then there's the fact that he was an emotional eater; his weight problems started when he was eight. It's possible, after all, to overeat even healthy foods; he used to overeat both the right and wrong stuff because he was distressed. He just hated exercise; he wouldn't mind me telling you this, but he used to cry at the gym and would call me the Daughter of Satan for pushing him to exercise.

Del had all of the typical struggles that obese people have. He had lost weight and gained it back, plateaued, gone back to emotional eating, eaten in secret, battled all of the demons associated with eating, and then set himself right again. But he never went back to animal foods. In all these years that he's been dealing with his weight, he never picked up a piece of cheese and he never had a chicken wing. He tended to overeat pretzels and beer and potato chips.

GM: So since he's been on your program, has he had these relapses?

PP: Oh, yeah. It's never a straight line to success. I think Del typifies a lot of people who struggle with food because their reasons for eating are different than yours and mine. I mean, I love food and I love to eat, but if I'm not hungry, I'm not going to go gorge on something. And if you make me angry, I'm more likely to skip lunch than eat two lunches. Del, on the other hand, has always anesthetized himself with food; he's had to learn new behaviors to not do it. And he's also had to learn to prioritize because when you don't like to exercise, it's the first thing that goes when you're busy. All your best habits go out the window. In the last year, he's gotten to the place where he disciplines himself all the more to stay with the right behaviors the busier he is.

I've told Del that an alcoholic always has to get up every morning and remember how to avoid alcohol, but you can't do that with food. That complicates the matter. An alcoholic is one drink away from disaster, and a drug addict is one pill away from disaster, but you can't say that a food addict is one calorie away from disaster. So every day you've got to get up and remember your strategies for not abusing food and not anesthetizing yourself with food. You always have to be mindful because that's the first place the demons inside you want to go. For an anorexic, the first place they want to go is starvation. For a food addict, the first place they want to go is overeating; that's how they deal with life, so every day you've got to be mindful. He's finally gotten to the place where it's not such a struggle. It will always be more of a struggle for him than for me, but it's not going to be like it used to be. So he's overcome, and I have a lot of respect for him. Plus, as a chef, he works with food and has it in front of him all day long.

GM: Has Del had other problems with his health that have gone away since he's lost weight?

PP: Yeah, he had gastroparesis. Del was a person who could eat breakfast at five in the morning and it would still be making him sick at eight in the morning—he might even throw it up. That completely went away.

128

GM: And does he still hate exercise?

Hummus

4 cups cooked garbanzo beans, warmed

3 cloves garlic

¼ cup lemon juice

2 teaspoons cumin powder

Sea salt to taste

Combine all ingredients in a blender and puree until smooth. Add water as needed to make a smooth paste. Serve with pita bread, crackers, or fresh vegetables.

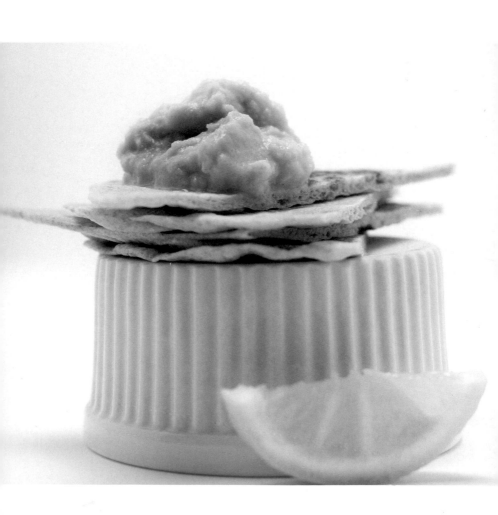

Miso Almond Spread

1 pound extra-firm tofu

6 tablespoons toasted almond butter

3 tablespoons mellow white miso

3 cloves garlic, minced

2 tablespoons fresh dill

½ medium red onion, minced

Place tofu, almond butter, miso, and garlic into a food processor. Blend until smooth and creamy. Remove the tofu mixture to a mixing bowl and add the remaining ingredients. Stir to combine.

Del's Big Green Salad

8 ounces mixed greens

1 cup garbanzo beans

1 cup red cabbage, grated

½ cup raisins

½ cup sunflower seeds, toasted

1 carrot, grated

Sweet and Spicy Mustard Dressing, recipe follows

Divide the mixed greens between four dinner plates. Arrange the remaining ingredients on top of the greens and serve with Sweet and Spicy Mustard Dressing on the side.

Sweet and Spicy Mustard Dressing

1 package silken tofu

½ cup prepared mustard

½ cup maple syrup

2 tablespoon lemon juice

½ teaspoon sea salt

¼ teaspoon cayenne pepper

Combine all ingredients in a food processor and puree until smooth and creamy.

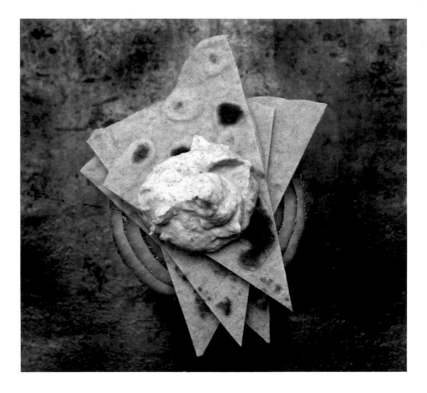

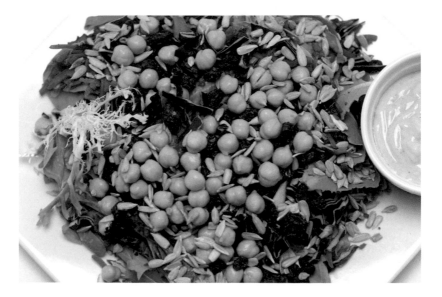

Potato Leek Soup

3 large leeks (about 1 pound),
thinly sliced

6 cups vegetable stock

4 or 5 medium russet potatoes
(1 pound), peeled and
chopped

¼ cup parsley, minced

¼ cup chives, minced

Sea salt and white pepper to
taste

Sauté the leeks over medium heat in a large stockpot, stirring occasionally, until the leeks have begun to soften and brown slightly, about eight minutes. Add water one to two tablespoons at a time, as needed, to prevent the leeks from sticking.

Add the vegetable stock and potatoes and bring to a boil over high heat. Reduce the heat to medium-low and simmer until the vegetables are tender, about 35 minutes.

Blend the soup until smooth using either an immersion blender or by carefully transferring the soup to a blender in batches.

Return the soup to the pot and add the parsley and chives. Cook five more minutes and season with salt and pepper. Serve immediately.

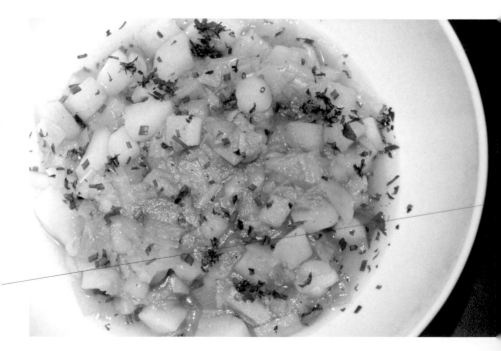

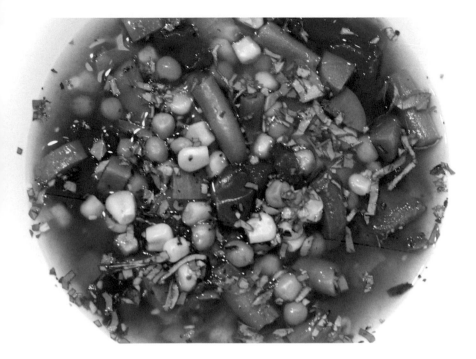

Tomato Vegetable Soup

SERVES 8 TO 10

2 large yellow onions, diced
   ½ inch

3 large carrots, diced ½ inch

3 stalks celery, diced ½ inch

6 cloves garlic, minced

1 tablespoon fresh thyme, minced

2 bay leaves

4 cups tomatoes, diced

1½ cups corn

1½ cups frozen green beans

1½ cups frozen peas

6 cups vegetable stock

1 cup basil, finely chopped

Sea salt and black pepper to
   taste

Sauté the onions, carrots, and celery until the onions are translucent, about seven to eight minutes. Add the garlic, thyme, and bay leaves; cook another minute. Add the tomatoes, corn, green beans, peas, and vegetable stock. Cook, covered, over medium heat for 20 to 25 minutes. Add the basil, season with salt and pepper, and cook another five minutes.

Black Bean Chili

SERVES 6 TO 8

2 medium yellow onions, diced

2 tablespoons garlic, minced

1½ tablespoons cumin

½ tablespoon dried sage

1 tablespoon chili powder

2 teaspoons oregano

2 green peppers, diced

4 cups cooked black beans

4 cups tomatoes, diced

3 cups vegetable broth

Sea salt and black pepper to taste

Sauté the onions in a large stockpot for eight minutes over medium heat. Add water one to two tablespoons at a time to keep the onions from sticking. Add the garlic, cumin, dried sage, chili powder, and oregano; cook one minute.

Add the remaining ingredients and cook, covered, for 20 minutes over medium heat. Season with salt and pepper; cook another five minutes.

Millet Loaf

SERVES 4

3½ cups water

1¾ cups millet

2 large leeks, diced small and rinsed

3 celery stalks, diced small

3 cloves garlic, minced

¼ cup fresh basil, minced

2 teaspoons fresh thyme leaves, minced

1 cup tomato sauce, divided

Bring the water to a boil in a medium saucepan. Add the millet and cook covered for 20 minutes.

Preheat the oven to 350 degrees.

Preheat a large skillet over medium heat and add the leek and celery. Sauté for eight or nine minutes, or until the leeks start to brown. Add water one to two tablespoons at a time, as needed, to keep the vegetables from sticking.

Add the garlic, basil, and thyme; cook another minute. Add half of the tomato sauce and the cooked millet. Mix well and spoon the mixture into a nonstick loaf pan. Top with the remaining tomato sauce and bake for 35 to 40 minutes.

Remove from the oven and let sit for 15 minutes before slicing.

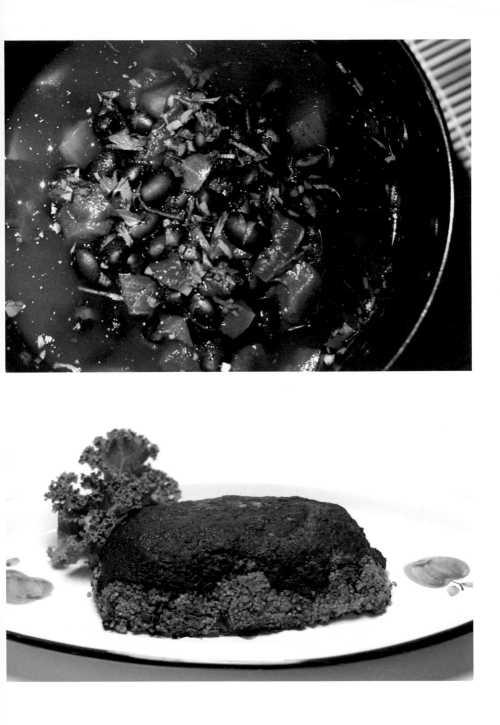

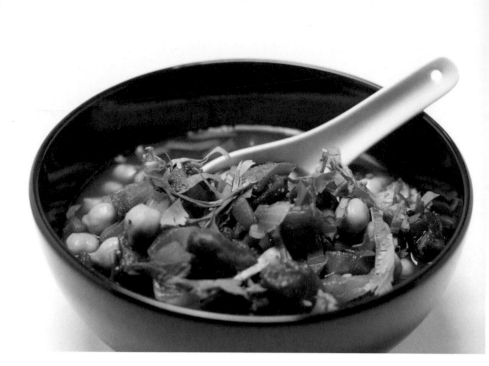

North African Chickpeas

SERVES 4

1 medium yellow onion, diced

1 green bell pepper, diced

3 garlic cloves, minced

2 teaspoons cumin

½ teaspoon turmeric

2 cups tomatoes, diced

3 cups cooked chickpeas

1 cup vegetable broth

1 pinch saffron steeped in hot
water for 15 minutes

Sea salt to taste

½ cup cilantro, chopped

Sauté the onion and green bell pepper in a large skillet over medium heat for seven to eight minutes. Add water one to two table-spoons at a time to keep the vegetables from sticking. Add the garlic, cumin, and turmeric. Cook another minute. Add the tomatoes, chick-peas, vegetable broth, and saffron, and cook 10 to 12 minutes. Season with sea salt to taste and cook another five minutes.

Serve garnished with the chopped cilantro.

Spring Vegetable Stir Fry

SERVES 2 TO 3

1 small yellow onion, thinly
   sliced

1 carrot, cut into matchsticks

½ bunch asparagus, trimmed
   and cut into 1-inch pieces

1 cup sugar snap peas,
   trimmed and cut in half

1 tablespoon fresh ginger,
   peeled and minced

3 cloves garlic, chopped

¼ cup toasted almonds,
   coarsely chopped

2 tablespoons hoisin sauce

¼ cup cilantro, chopped

¼ cup chives, chopped

Sea salt to taste

Heat a large skillet over high heat. Add the onion and carrot; stir fry three minutes. Add water one to two tablespoons at a time to keep the vegetables from sticking. Add the asparagus and sugar snap peas; cook two minutes. Add the remaining ingredients and cook three minutes longer.

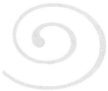

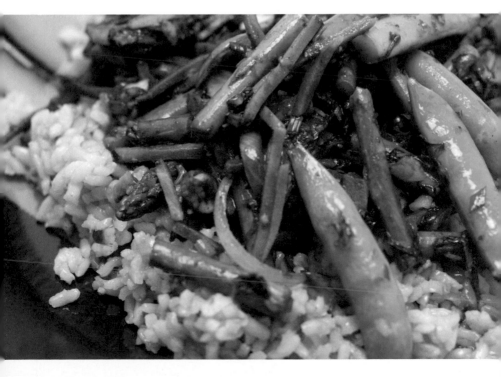

Quinoa Pilaf

SERVES 4

1 medium yellow onion, diced

2 stalks celery, diced

1 medium green bell pepper, diced

2 cloves garlic, minced

1 teaspoon fresh sage, minced

1 teaspoon fresh thyme, minced

One 28-ounce can diced tomatoes

1 cup vegetable broth

1 cup quinoa, rinsed and drained

Sea salt and black pepper to taste

Sauté the onion, celery, and green bell pepper in a large saucepan for five minutes. Add water one to two tablespoons at a time to keep them from sticking. Add the garlic, sage, and thyme; cook another minute. Add the tomatoes, vegetable broth, and quinoa; bring to a boil over high heat. Cover the pan, reduce the heat to medium, and cook the pilaf until the quinoa is tender, about 15 to 20 minutes. Season with salt and black pepper.

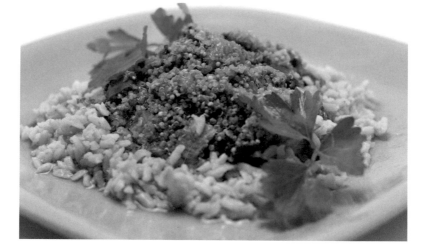

Lentil Cakes

SERVES 6

3½ cups vegetable stock

1½ cups green lentils

2 medium leeks, diced small and cleaned

Combine the vegetable stock and lentils in a medium stockpot and bring to a boil over high heat. Cover the pot, reduce the heat to medium, and cook the lentils until tender, about 45 to 50 minutes.

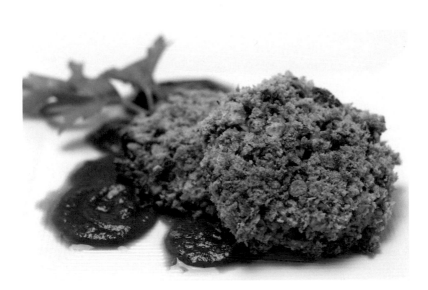

1 large carrot, diced small

2 celery stalks, diced small

2 teaspoons fresh thyme, minced

2 cloves garlic, minced

Sea salt and black pepper

1 tablespoon arrowroot powder

2 cups whole grain bread crumbs, divided

While the lentils are cooking, sauté the leeks, carrot, and celery in a large saucepan over medium heat for 8 to 10 minutes. Add water one to two tablespoons at a time to keep the vegetables from sticking. Add the thyme and garlic; cook another minute. Set aside until the lentils are finished cooking.

When the lentils are tender, drain any excess liquid from the pan and let the lentils cool to room temperature. Mash the lentils just enough so that some of the texture remains in them. Add them to a bowl with the vegetable mixture, arrowroot powder, one cup of the bread crumbs, and salt and black pepper to taste. Mix well.

Divide the lentil mixture into 12 parts and shape each part into a half-inch-thick cake. Dredge each cake in the remaining bread crumbs and place each on a nonstick baking sheet. Bake the cakes for 20 minutes, turn them over, and bake another 20 minutes, or until browned.

Pierogies

Dough

2 cups semolina flour

1 teaspoon salt

¾ to 1 cup cold water

Combine the flour and salt in a medium mixing bowl. Add three-fourths cup water and mix it into the flour. Knead the dough. If it is dry, add more water—you should have a firm but pliable dough. Continue kneading for five minutes. Shape the dough into a ball and wrap in plastic wrap. Set the dough aside while you make the filling.

Filling

2 medium russet potatoes, scrubbed, peeled, and diced

1 teaspoon granulated onion

Sea salt to taste

Add the potatoes to a medium saucepan and cover with cold water. Bring the pan to a boil over high heat. Cover the pan, reduce the heat to a simmer, and cook the potatoes until tender, about 12 to 15 minutes. Drain off all but one-fourth cup of the cooking liquid, add the granulated onion and sea salt to taste, and mash the potatoes.

Caramelized Onions

2 large yellow onions, diced small

Add the onions to a large saucepan and cook over medium heat for about 15 minutes, or until the onions are well browned. Add water one to two tablespoons at a time to keep the onions from sticking. Set the cooked onions aside while you prepare the rest of the dish.

Horseradish Sauce

1 package silken tofu

1 tablespoon, more or less to taste, prepared horseradish

Sea salt to taste

Combine all ingredients in a blender and puree until smooth and creamy.

TO ASSEMBLE AND COOK THE PIEROGIES

Divide the dough into two parts. Roll one half of the dough until one-eighth-inch thick. Cut circles with a three-inch cookie cutter. Add a teaspoon or so of filling to the center of each circle. Fold the circles in half over the filling and pinch closed. Make sure the seams are airtight so they don't burst open when cooking. Set each pierogi on a flour-dusted cookie sheet while you prepare the rest of them. Roll out the other half of the dough, then cut, fill, and seal.

To cook the pierogies, bring a pot of water to a boil and salt it. Add the pierogies one at a time and boil them for four minutes, or until they float.

Add the cooked pierogies to the pan with the caramelized onions, season with salt and pepper, and serve with horseradish sauce.

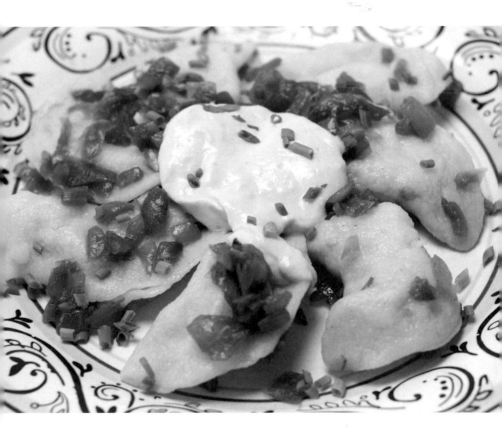

Sweet and Sour Tofu

SERVES 4

1 pound extra-firm tofu, drained

¼ cup Bragg Liquid Aminos

¼ cup maple syrup

3 cloves garlic, minced

2 tablespoons fresh ginger, minced

Black pepper to taste

1 cup Sweet and Sour Sauce, recipe follows

Preheat the oven to 350 degrees.

Cut the tofu into three-fourths-inch cubes. Place the cubes on a small baking sheet (the smaller the better so all of the marinade will absorb into the tofu). Set aside while you prepare the marinade.

Combine all the ingredients for the marinade and pour over the tofu mixture. Let sit for one hour.

Bake for 20 minutes. Turn and bake another 20 minutes. Remove the tofu from the baking sheet into a bowl and add the sauce. Toss to mix well.

Sweet and Sour Sauce

1½ cups apple cider or apple juice

¼ cup cider vinegar

¼ cup Bragg Liquid Aminos

¼ cup plus 2 tablespoons maple syrup

1 garlic clove, minced

2 tablespoons arrowroot powder

Combine everything in a saucepan and whisk to mix well. Bring the mixture to a boil over high heat and let cook one minute until thickened.

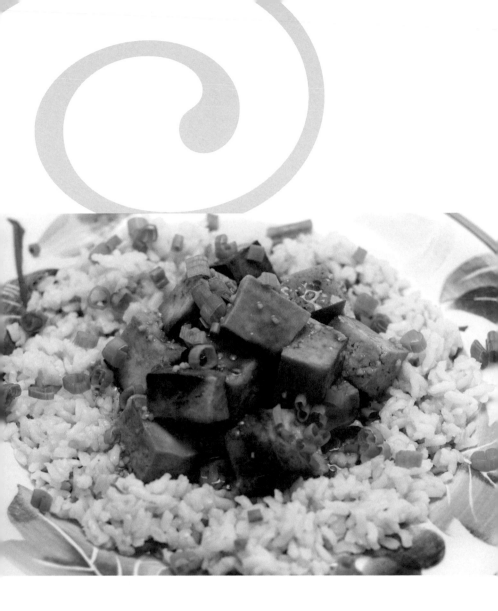

Barbecue Tofu

SERVES 4

1 pound of extra-firm tofu, drained, rinsed, and patted dry

3 tablespoons unsweetened almond milk mixed with 1 tablespoon arrowroot powder

3 tablespoons whole wheat pastry flour

3 tablespoons nutritional yeast

1½ tablespoons granulated garlic

1 teaspoon sea salt

1⅓ cups Barbecue Sauce, recipe follows

Preheat oven to 350 degrees.

Cut the tofu into three-fourths-inch cubes. Place cubes in a large bowl and toss with the almond milk mixture. In a separate bowl, combine the remaining ingredients. Add to the bowl with the tofu and toss gently to coat the tofu.

Place on a nonstick baking sheet and bake for 20 minutes. Turn the tofu and bake another 20 minutes.

To assemble, combine the prepared oven-fried tofu and one cup sauce in a mixing bowl. Stir to combine well.

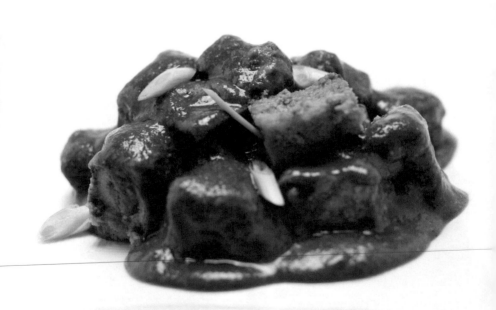

Barbecue Sauce

1 medium yellow onion, diced small

2 cloves garlic, minced

2 cups tomato sauce

Zest and juice of 1 orange

½ cup maple syrup

1 tablespoon molasses

½ cup prepared mustard

1 teaspoon allspice

1 tablespoon Bragg Liquid Aminos

Sauté the onion in a large saucepan over medium heat for 10 minutes. Add water one to two tablespoons at a time to keep the onion from sticking. Add the garlic and cook another minute.

Add the remaining ingredients and cook for 20 minutes.

Caribbean "Chicken" and Olives

SERVES 4

1 medium yellow onion, diced small

½ teaspoon dried thyme

1 clove garlic, minced

One 18-ounce package "Chicken"-style seitan, minced

4 green onions, sliced

¼ cup seedless raisins, soaked in warm water for 10 minutes and drained

Crushed red pepper

¼ cup vegetable stock

4 cups cooked brown rice

Sauté the onion over medium heat for eight minutes. Add water one to two tablespoons at a time to keep the onion from sticking. Add the thyme and garlic; cook another minute. Add the seitan, green onion, raisins, crushed red pepper to taste, and one-fourth cup vegetable stock. Cook for five minutes. Serve over the brown rice.

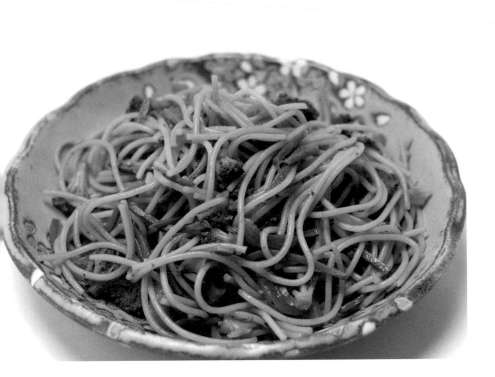

Vegetable Chow Mein

SERVES 2

8 ounces brown rice noodles, cooked according to package instructions

¼ cup **Bragg Liquid Aminos**

3 tablespoons maple syrup

2 cloves garlic, minced

1 teaspoon ginger, minced

1 small yellow onion, cut into thin slices

1 carrot, julienned

2 cups small broccoli florets

Cook the brown rice noodles. While the pasta cooks, combine the Bragg Liquid Aminos, maple syrup, garlic, and ginger in a small bowl and set aside.

Heat a large skillet over high heat. Add the onion and carrot; stir-fry for three to four minutes. Add water one to two tablespoons at a time to keep the vegetables from sticking. Add the broccoli and cook for five minutes, adding more water as needed.

When the vegetables are tender, add the Bragg Liquid Aminos mixture and cook another minute. Add the cooked noodles and mix well.

Spinach Enchiladas

½ pound extra-firm tofu

1 package silken tofu

2 tablespoons nut yeast

1 medium yellow onion, diced small

3 cloves garlic, minced

1 tablespoon cumin

1 tablespoon chili powder

Sea salt and black pepper to taste

One 10-ounce package frozen spinach, thawed, wrung dry, and chopped

12 corn tortillas

2 cups Enchilada Sauce, recipe follows

Mash the extra-firm tofu and silken tofu in a mixing bowl using a potato masher. Add the nutritional yeast and set aside.

Sauté the onion over medium heat in a large skillet for eight minutes. Add water one to two tablespoons at a time to keep the onion from sticking. Add the garlic, cumin, and chili powder; cook another minute.

Add the onion mixture and spinach to the mashed tofu and set aside.

Heat the corn tortillas until softened, a few at a time, in a large skillet over medium heat. Place each on a flat surface and put three to four tablespoons of the spinach filling down the middle of the tortilla. Roll up the tortilla around the filling and place it seam side down in a 9x13-inch baking dish. Repeat until all of the tortillas are used up.

Pour the sauce over the enchiladas and bake for 20 minutes.

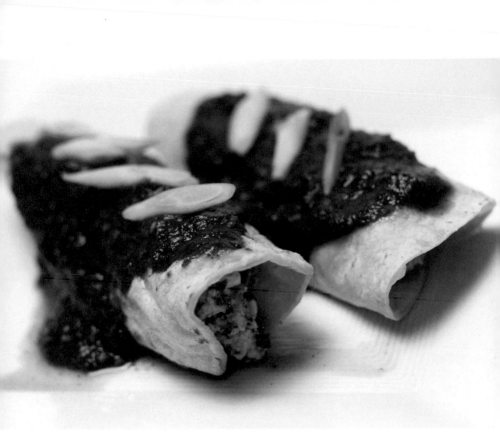

Enchilada Sauce

MAKES 2 CUPS

1 small yellow onion, diced

1 teaspoon cumin

2 teaspoons oregano

2 garlic cloves, minced

One 15-ounce can diced
   tomatoes

2 ancho chiles in adobo sauce

Saute the onion over medium heat for 10 minutes. Add water one to two tablespoons at a time to keep the onion from sticking. Add the cumin, oregano, and garlic; cook another minute.

Puree the tomatoes with the ancho chiles in adobo sauce; add puree to the pan.

Cook over medium-low heat for 20 minutes. Taste for salt.

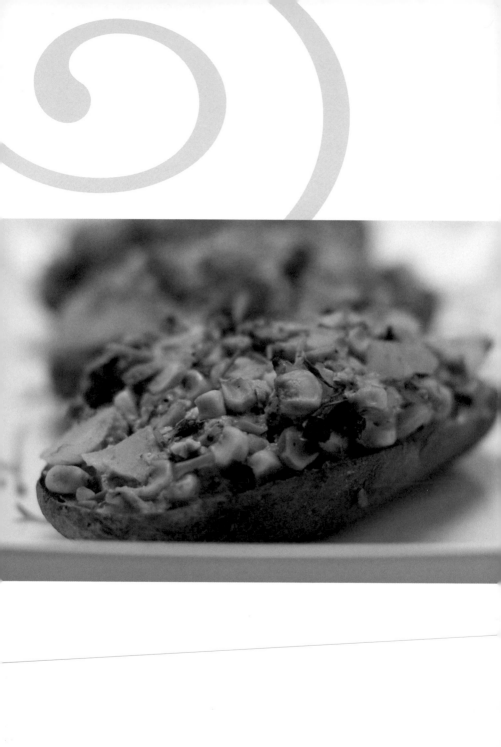

Twice-Baked Potatoes

SERVES 6

6 large russet potatoes

1 medium yellow onion, diced

1 red bell pepper, diced

Corn cut from 4 ears (about 3 cups)

1 large head broccoli, cut into small florets

1 medium zucchini, quartered lengthwise and thinly sliced

3 cloves garlic, minced

1 package silken tofu, pureed

½ cup nutritional yeast

Sea salt and black pepper to taste

Preheat oven to 350 degrees.

Scrub the potatoes and wrap them individually in aluminum foil. Place them on a nonstick baking sheet and cook for one hour, or until tender. Remove potatoes from the oven and set aside while you prepare the filling.

Sauté the onion, red bell pepper, and corn in a large skillet over medium-high heat for six to eight minutes, or until the vegetables start to turn brown. Add water one to two tablespoons at a time to keep the vegetables from sticking. Add the broccoli and cook, covered, for another five minutes. Add the zucchini and cook until tender, about three to four minutes. Add the garlic, season with salt and pepper, and add the pureed tofu and nutritional yeast.

When the potatoes are cool enough to handle, cut a slit lengthwise down the middle of each potato. Squeeze it open and scoop out most of the innards, leaving a half-inch wall. Coarsely chop the scooped potato and add it to the cooked vegetable filling.

Divide the filling evenly between each of the potatoes and return to the baking sheet. Cook for 20 minutes, or until the potatoes are hot.

Stir Fry Pasta with Vegetables

SERVES 4

12 ounces whole grain penne pasta, cooked according to package instructions

½ medium yellow onion, julienned

1 medium carrot, cut into matchsticks

1 large head broccoli, cut into florets

1 cup sugar snap peas, ends trimmed and cut in half

3 cloves garlic, minced

2 teaspoons fresh ginger, minced

3 tablespoons Bragg Liquid Aminos, more or less to taste

Black pepper to taste

Cook the pasta. Heat a large skillet over high heat. Add the onion, carrots, and broccoli. Stir-fry for four minutes, adding water one to two tablespoons at a time to keep the vegetables from sticking. Add the sugar snap peas and cook for two minutes. Add the garlic, ginger, Bragg Liquid Aminos, and cooked pasta. Cook another minute and season with black pepper.

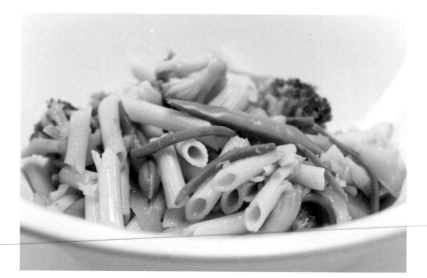

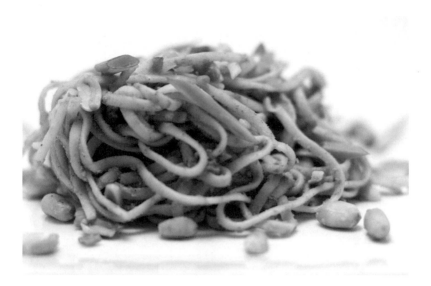

Spicy Thai Peanut Noodles

SERVES 4 TO 6

12 cloves garlic, minced

¼ cup fresh ginger, minced

1 jalapeño pepper, minced

1 tablespoon ground ginger

½ tablespoon cayenne pepper

½ cup Bragg Liquid Aminos

2 tablespoons red wine vinegar

¼ cup plus 2 tablespoons cane sugar

¾ cup water

1 cup peanut butter

1 pound linguine, cooked according to package instructions

½ bunch green onions, thinly sliced

1 medium cucumber, halved, seeded, and thinly sliced

For the peanut sauce, combine the garlic, ginger, jalapeño pepper, ground ginger, cayenne pepper, Bragg Liquid Aminos, vinegar, sugar, and water in a large pot; bring the mixture to a boil. Let cook one minute and remove the pot from heat. Add the peanut butter and whisk to combine well.

While the sauce is cooking, prepare the pasta.

Drain the pasta and add it to a bowl with the sauce. Mix well. Serve garnished with green onions and cucumber slices.

Thai Pizza

MAKES ONE 12-INCH PIZZA

One prebaked, 12-inch whole grain pizza crust

½ cup peanut sauce (see Spicy Thai Peanut Noodles)

1 cup snow peas, sliced on a diagonal

1 cup green onion, sliced

1 medium tomato, diced

1 cup mung bean sprouts

¼ cup toasted peanuts

½ cup basil, chopped

Preheat the oven to 375 degrees.

Spread the peanut sauce over the crust and top with snow peas, green onion, and tomato. Place the pizza on a baking sheet and cook for 12 to 13 minutes. Remove from the oven and top with the sprouts, basil, and peanuts.

Del's Favorite Pizza

MAKES ONE 12-INCH PIZZA

One prebaked, 12-inch whole grain pizza crust

½ cup tomato sauce, more or less to taste

½ green bell pepper, diced

1 cup mushrooms, sliced

½ cup red onion, diced

½ batch oven-fried tofu (use recipe for Barbecue Tofu, without sauce)

Fresh basil for garnish

Preheat the oven to 375 degrees.

Place the pizza crust on a baking sheet and spread the tomato sauce over it. Top with the remaining ingredients and bake for 13 to 14 minutes. Garnish with the fresh basil.

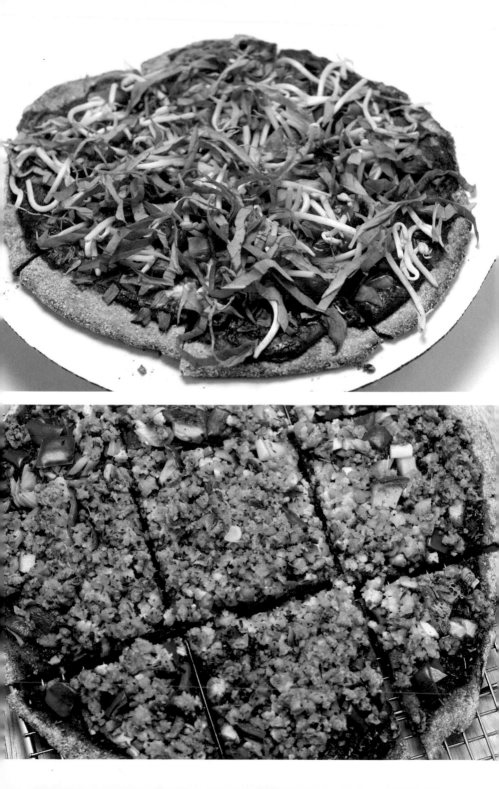

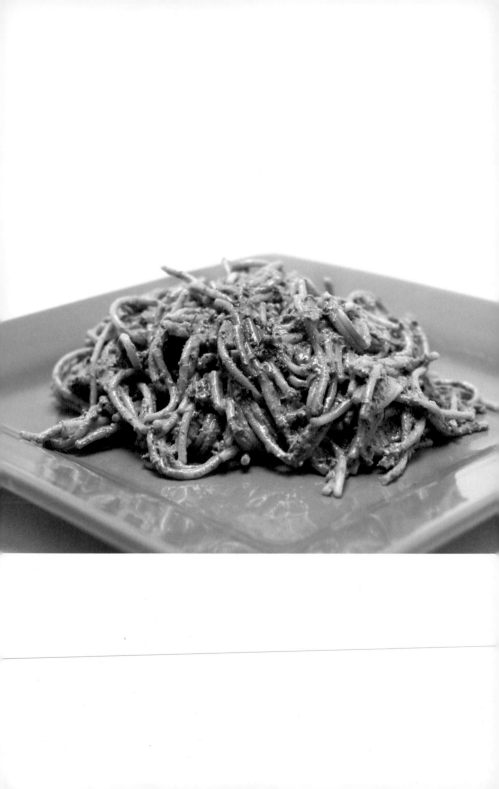

Pesto Pasta

SERVES 4 TO 6

1 pound whole grain linguine

1 cup Creamy Basil Pesto,
recipe follows

Cook the pasta according to package instructions, then drain it, reserving one-fourth cup of the liquid.

Add the cooked pasta and pesto to a large bowl and mix well.

Creamy Basil Pesto

2 cups fresh basil leaves,
packed

½ package silken tofu

¼ cup nutritional yeast

¼ cup walnuts, toasted

2 cloves garlic, chopped

Sea salt and black pepper to
taste

Combine everything in the bowl of a food processor and puree until smooth and creamy.

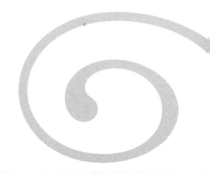

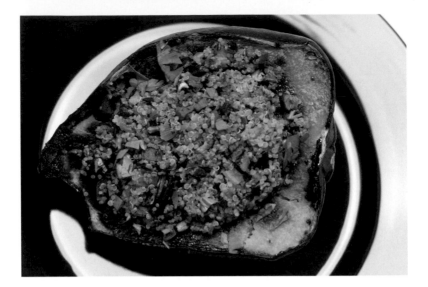

Stuffed Baked Squash

2 acorn squash, halved and seeded

Sea salt to taste

1½ cups vegetable broth

¾ cup quinoa, rinsed and drained

1 medium onion, diced small

1 stalk celery, diced small

1 medium carrot, diced small

2 cloves garlic, minced

1 teaspoon fresh thyme, minced

1 teaspoon sage, minced

Salt and black pepper to taste

¾ cup pecans, toasted 7 to 8 minutes in a 350-degree oven

Preheat oven to 350 degrees.

Cut both acorn squash in half crosswise; remove seeds and fibers. Sprinkle salt over cut halves. Place halves in a shallow nonstick baking pan. Add one cup water to the pan. Bake for about 40 minutes, or until tender.

While the squash bakes, prepare the stuffing.

In heavy saucepan, bring broth to a boil. Add the quinoa and cover the pan. Bring it to a boil over high heat and then reduce heat to medium low. Let simmer for 20 minutes, or until the quinoa is tender.

Sauté the onion, celery, and carrot for seven minutes over medium heat. Add the garlic, thyme, sage, salt, and pepper; cook another minute. Remove from heat; fold in the pecans and cooked quinoa.

Spoon the quinoa mixture into the baked squash. Cover with foil, return to the oven, and bake another 20 minutes.

Dr. Pam's Vanilla Ice "Cream"

SERVES 1

2 whole bananas, peeled, sliced, and frozen

¼ cup unsweetened almond milk

¼ teaspoon vanilla extract

1 packet stevia or more to taste

Combine all ingredients in a food processor or blender with a powerful motor, and process until the ice cream is smooth and creamy.

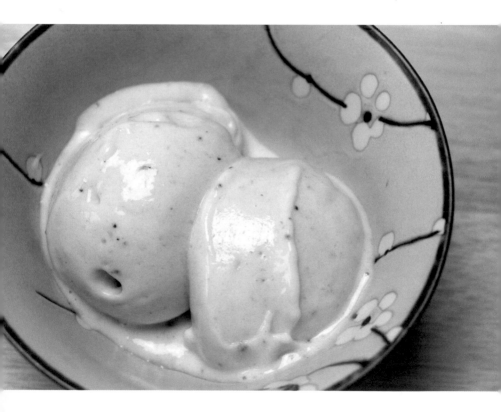

Fruit Crisp

9 cups (about 2 pounds) pears, cored, peeled, and sliced

¼ cup organic cane sugar

2 tablespoons fresh lemon juice

1 teaspoon cinnamon

¼ teaspoon nutmeg

Topping

1 cup rolled oats, regular or quick-cooking

½ cup whole wheat pastry flour

½ cup organic cane sugar

1 teaspoon cinnamon

¼ cup plus 2 tablespoons unsweetened applesauce

Preheat the oven to 350 degrees.

In a large bowl, combine the pears, sugar, lemon juice, one teaspoon cinnamon, and nutmeg. Mix well and transfer the mixture into a 9x13-inch nonstick baking dish.

In a medium bowl, combine the oats, flour, sugar, and one teaspoon cinnamon. Add the applesauce and mix well.

Sprinkle topping over pear mixture. Bake for 50 minutes, or until topping is nicely browned on top.

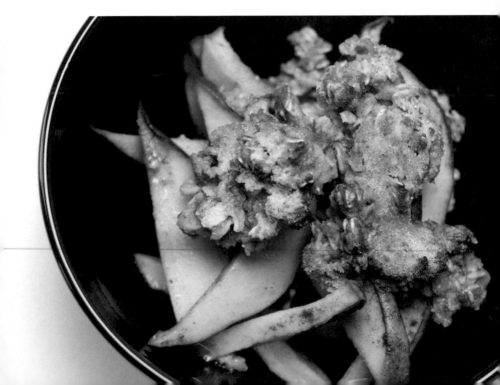

PP: Not as much. He bitches and moans about it, but he basically enjoys the gym. He likes being fit and he likes the way it makes him feel. He now notices that you feel better when you do it than when you don't. And sometimes you dread it the most when you need it the most. I've dragged my butt into yoga sometimes when I think I'm going to die, but that's when I need to go more than ever.

GM: I'm still trying to picture the scene when this guy comes in at 475 pounds and you decide to make him a partner in Wellness Forum Foods.

PP: With two caveats. The two rules when he joined us were: One, he had to lose the weight. Two, he had to take the oils out of the food.

GM: And his response?

PP: He agreed, but he said, "Pammy, I'll do a lot of things but I'm not giving up taste." I said, "Well, you don't have to give up the taste; just figure out how to do it without the fat." And his food is amazing. This guy is amazing.

Now, Del already had a business. He had a large clientele of people for whom he was making food on a regular basis.

GM: A meal-delivery service?

PP: Right. We bought the delivery service and moved Del into the building. And he was nervous about one thing. He said, "Well, Pammy, what are we going to tell all these people I've been cooking for all these years when the oil comes out of the food?" I said, "Well, how about this: Why don't we just not say anything? And then if someone complains, we'll explain the health benefits of eating without oil." This was back in 2005. And not one

FOOD OVER MEDICINE

person ever said anything about the missing oil. Well, actually no, I shouldn't say that. One person said, "Hey, Del, since you got hooked up with Wellness Forum, your food isn't as greasy anymore!" The other three hundred people never noticed anything at all; they've never commented about it.

GM: So he kept the same clients and they didn't even notice the changes?

PP: Exactly. So there's another reason to get the oil out of the diet: not only is it high in fat and calories and contributory to cardiovascular disease but it's also completely unnecessary; there is absolutely no reason to include it. We've never shown somebody how to make food without oil who three months later was saying, "Gosh, I really miss the oil. If only I could have some oil on my pasta dish, life would be fine." None of them say that; they just don't care about it. If you don't miss it when it's gone, if it doesn't change how fabulous the food is, and if it's detrimental to your health, then why include it? Del has become a master at showing people how to cook without added fat.

DEL SROUFE IN HIS OWN WORDS

My weight problems started as a child. I remember being put on a diet of only eight hundred calories per day when I was only eight years old. I overate and my mother dealt with that by helping me to control portion size. It didn't work; my weight problems carried over into adulthood.

Several years ago, I started my own business, a vegan bakery, and converted to vegan eating at that time. I had previously worked in a "health food" restaurant, which I later learned was not so healthy after all. That is where my consumption of vegan junk food really began.

Believe it or not, I gained one hundred pounds within one year of starting my bakery, and the weight gain continued until I peaked at 475 pounds. You might be wondering how an individual consuming a vegan diet could accomplish this. Here's how I did it.

Every day I started my day with two fresh scones and coffee. Then, I proceeded to eat a cashew bar and muffin for lunch, or cake, or whatever was handy—I was working very hard and rarely sat down to eat a full meal. I continued to munch on sugary foods and drink caffeine-filled beverages throughout the day and for "real meals," I would eat vegetarian foods prepared with lots of oil and fat. In the evenings, to relax, I'd eat potato chips and drink beer. All vegan, but certainly not healthy.

In the summer of 2005, I reached my wit's end. I was exhausted. My body ached, my knees ached. I fell and my injured ankle would not heal. I needed help.

I went to my good friend Dr. Pam Popper and told her I was ready to change my life! I immediately converted to a well-structured plant-based diet; instead of scones and coffee for breakfast, I started having fruit smoothies and whole-grain cereal. I replaced my constant snacking with meals comprised of beans, whole grains, potatoes, and salads. And the weight started coming off right away.

I lost fifty pounds in the first six months and hit a plateau, at which time Dr. Pam told me I had to start moving. I started walking, since that was the least painful thing I could do. The weight started dropping again.

(cont'd. on next page)

(cont'd. from previous page)

At seventy-five pounds, I hit another plateau, and the advice was to step up the exercise. This is when I started working out with Dr. Pam and taking Wellness Forum hot yoga classes. And that is when the weight started dropping like crazy. People started telling me I looked different almost from day to day. I must confess that stepping up the exercise program was the most miserable thing I have ever done in my life. I used to hiss at Dr. Pam in the gym, and lay on my yoga mat praying for death. Fortunately, this did not last long, and although I hated to admit it, I started to enjoy getting into shape. I actually missed working out when my schedule caused me to miss a day.

I still have another thirty pounds to lose, but it's getting easier and easier every day. I don't even have to think about things most days. I just eat the way I've formed the habit of eating, do the required exercise, and the weight comes off.

Here's the best part—I'm working harder than I've ever worked in my life and I'm less tired as a result of doing it. My ankle is finally healing. I'm wearing clothes that I haven't worn for years. I feel great about myself. I may even run a marathon with Dr. Pam now that I have all of this energy.

So, let me emphasize a couple of things. First, conversion to a vegan diet does not, in and of itself, lead to health. You have to convert to a well-structured vegan diet. I have quit sabotaging myself—the wrong foods are like drugs for me— and when I think about not eating healthfully, I remember my goals and I don't eat them. I am learning to make self-care a priority; no matter how busy I am, I make time to eat good food and to exercise. And I try to be around like-minded people who reinforce my good habits.

I have no desire to return to the way I used to be.

PAM'S NOTE: Del will never return to the way he used to be because he now understands and follows the dietary principles that will prevent a slide back into obesity. Meanwhile, his recipes have helped thousands of others enjoy meals created according to those same guidelines, especially now through his bestselling *Forks Over Knives—The Cookbook* and his forthcoming *Better Than Vegan*. The insert section in this book contains a never-before-published sampling of some of Del's favorite recipes that we use here at The Wellness Forum, and that everyone loves.

THE DIETARY
ESTABLISHMENT

. . . .

GM: Pam, I just went on the website of the Academy of Nutrition and Dietetics (AND). I clicked on "nutrition for growing bodies" and saw that they recommend whole grains, fruits, and veggies, including 100 percent juice, low-fat dairy foods, and then a protein group that is lean meat, poultry, fish, eggs, beans, and nuts.

PP: Right. Hey, it's the dietary recommendations of the United States Department of Agriculture (USDA). If the USDA issued recommendations tomorrow for everyone to drink ten ounces of arsenic before breakfast, it'd be posted on AND's website by noon.

GM: Ha!

PP: I'm not kidding! And this stuff is important because these are the people providing the dietary guidelines that are being used to design school lunches.

GM: I read in the *New York Times* about a study that showed that children who eat school lunches are 29 percent more likely to be obese than kids who bring their own lunches to school.[1]

PP: And since their own lunches probably aren't so great, that gives you an idea of just how awful the school lunches are. The Physicians Committee for Responsible Medicine (PCRM) filed a lawsuit against the USDA over the latest dietary guidelines because they're so horrific. Not only does AND not say that the guidelines are terrible but its president issued a press release gushing about what a great job the USDA committee did and how hard it worked to sort through all this science to come up with this wonderful recommendation. The president also reminded us, by the way, that AND is the group of people you want to look to for dietary information.[2] It's almost like the USDA has put AND on the payroll, which wouldn't be surprising because everyone else has. If the USDA isn't paying AND, then that would be the one group that has somehow been exempted.

GM: What do you mean by that? Who's paying AND?

PP: They're heavily funded by sponsors. Millions of dollars a year.

GM: The dairy industry?

PP: Oh, there aren't any that are missed. The dairy industry, the beef industry, food manufacturers like Wrigley and Hershey's and Kellogg's—there's no discernment. If you own a food company and you want to sponsor AND, just step up to the plate with your wallet open. There's no filtering that says you have to qualify based on promoting a healthful food.[3] So the American Distillers Association, the lamb industry, there's nobody exempt from their endorsement, provided they show up with a check.

GM: Is there no group of critics within AND, no group of dietitians, that fights this system and calls it corrupt?

PP: Not within AND. You have the same thing going on with dietitians that you have going on with medical doctors. When we talk about how bad health care is and how corrupt the medical system is, it all starts with corrupt professional organizations. Just as Dr. John McDougall is not representative of the medical profession, there are great dietitians out there, some of whom are close friends of mine, who have gone to dietetics school and held their noses in order to get their degrees. They've reengineered themselves to practice completely differently, to oppose within their own practice the guidelines of their umbrella organization. But there's no force within AND that is trying to change the system. Of course, AND's public stance is that it can't function without this type of money. How would the organization operate, after all? Of course, my response is that we've found a way to operate here and not take money from any corporate sponsors. If AND sends representatives, I'll show them how to do it with something interesting called earned income.

GM: Why couldn't AND function just on the dues of practicing members, rather than funds from corporate sponsors?

PP: Or selling services. There's no reason why AND couldn't actually market services in some ways directly to the public, but it's easier just to take the corporate bucks. I don't mean to pick on AND, because the American Academy of Pediatrics, the American Medical Association (AMA), and the American Diabetes

Association (ADA) all do it. They're all on the take. They're *all* taking money. It's pervasive in the health care business. So we have terrible recommendations that come from the federal government, and all of these organizations are corrupted by the same monetary influence.

GM: Who gives money, for example, to the AMA?

PP: The drug industry, mainly in the form of advertising in its journal. The American Psychiatric Association sends its journal free to its members. Guess how it gets to do that? Drug ads. Most of what psychiatrists are seeing is material promoted by the drug companies. I'd like to think that the average psychiatrist is smart enough to know that. Are they smart enough to say, "Maybe I should automatically be skeptical of anything these ads say that are printed in these journals?" I don't know. Psychiatrists are pretty drug-happy these days.

GM: Who gives money to the ADA?

PP: Well, the "health tip of the day" on the website was sponsored by Eskimo Pie for about eighteen months. Because if you're diabetic, you can never get enough Eskimo Pie.

The artificial sweetener companies contribute a lot. Cadbury Schweppes gave the ADA $1.5 million a few years ago. Cadbury is the third-largest maker of soft drinks in the world and also makes those crème eggs available at Easter. Those are some great items for diabetics also!

GM: Let me try to wrap my head around this. You're a manufacturer of soft drinks and you say, "Uh-oh, millions of people in America have become diabetic. That's not good for us because, after all, we're selling flavored sugar water. Here's an idea. Let's give money to the American Diabetes Association so that doctors won't tell their patients that soft drinks are bad for them?" Is that really conceivable?

PP: Well, they basically want the ADA to make mushy, meaningless pronouncements, which it faithfully does, as does the Academy of Nutrition and Dietetics. The party line that AND proudly announces to the general public is that there is room for everything in a healthy diet; that everything in moderation is fine; that there aren't any good and bad foods; that there aren't any good and bad dietary patterns; and that different things are appropriate for different people. And essentially it promotes this whole idea that sure, you can go ahead and have that soft drink with that Eskimo Pie.

I did a television interview recently in which this was a big topic of conversation. The promotion of this idea that you can just eat whatever you want without consequences. "You maybe want to do a little less of that and a little bit more of this, but nothing you eat is clearly right or wrong." You'll see a lot of statements from the American Diabetes Association, for example, to the effect that it's important to look at the whole range of products available to diabetics. Look at all the sugar-free drink products you can have, for example, if you're a little more sugar sensitive than somebody else. And the beverage industry is doing a great job by developing artificially sweetened soft drinks so that diabetics can enjoy these products, too. Yay! Now, of course, my employees here at The Wellness Forum joke that they've got guaranteed lifetime employment as long as this nonsense is going on, but I don't really think that's our objective here. I'd be happy to find something else to do with myself if we could fix the country's health problems.

GM: Let's talk about AND's recommendation to eat lean meat and poultry and fish and eggs. What is AND's factual basis for

139

this? I know that you make your dietary recommendations based on science. Maybe it's asking too much to expect AND to do the same, but is there any medical literature anywhere that suggests that there's anything healthy about poultry? Has there ever been a study done that if you eat poultry, it's good for any of your organs or has a positive effect on longevity? Is there any study in the world that suggests that poultry has health benefits?

PP: No.

GM: So no study has ever been done that eating poultry is any better for you than eating rice or beans or lentils or broccoli?

PP: No. We have studies that show the contrary.[4]

First, chicken contains just about as much fat as beef. Even chicken breast with the skin removed, and is broiled rather than fried, derives 23 percent of its calories from fat. And four ounces of chicken contains almost one hundred milligrams of cholesterol, about the same as four ounces of beef. And a study conducted by the Physicians Committee for Responsible Medicine determined that almost half of chicken sold in grocery stores was contaminated with feces.[5] Yet Americans have been told that chicken is better for them than beef and pork. This has caused chicken consumption to more than quadruple between 1950 and 2007, while beef consumption increased by only 50 percent and pork consumption went down.[6] Of course, Americans have continued to get fatter and sicker all the time.

GM: Well, is there any study that makes any positive case at all for poultry? Is there any study that shows that eating poultry is at least better for you than eating lizards, horses, chipmunks, or rats?

PP: No.

GM: So they're just pulling these recommendations out of their ass?

PP: They would clearly recommend the nutritional benefits of eating rats if there were a rat farm lobby or if people found fried rats delicious and there was a chain of Kentucky Fried Rat restaurants.

GM: Is it fair to say that a group like AND will promote some information occasionally that's based on science, and then other information—like advising people to eat lean meat and fish and eggs and poultry—that's just a safe way of endorsing the status quo, affirming the general culture and the standard American diet, without any science involved at all so as not to ruffle any feathers in, say, the poultry industry?

PP: Yes. And what makes this confusing to the general public is that people get on the AND website and, first of all, they have no idea how dietitians are trained and they assume the best. Then they see messages that are clearly right: eat more fruits and vegetables. I mean, who really disagrees with that? Whole grains and beans are good for you. So they see some things that are right and it makes them think this organization is probably right across the board. Even when there's clearly a sponsorship relationship, such as in the position papers. (It's printed in very small type in the website's right-hand corner.) I doubt the average person knows that the paper was written specifically in response to sponsorship money. The Wrigley Science Foundation sponsored a piece that stated you could add enamel to your teeth by chewing gum. Now, I have a lot of friends who are dentists and I've asked all of them, "What do you think of this?" They laugh out loud and say, "Who gave you that crazy idea?" Well, it was posted on AND's website.

The average person can't be expected to factor in the conflicts of interest. All the average person sees is that these organizations appear to be authoritative and the experts in the field. If you know no more than that, following their advice seems like the sensible thing to do.

GM: How about the governmental organizations? Do you feel the same way about the Food and Drug Administration (FDA) as you feel about these medical associations?

PP: Oh, it's probably worse.

GM: Then let's talk about the FDA.

PP: There are a few different issues to discuss: drug approval and regulation, and regulation of supplements, fortified foods, and the functional foods industry. In terms of the FDA's drug regulation, the flaw is that the drug companies make a lot of the decisions about study design, even about what's considered a side effect; they negotiate with the FDA on what should be listed as a side effect.

GM: How do you negotiate on what should be listed as a side effect?

PP: Well, Prozac doesn't list withdrawal symptoms as a side effect because both the manufacturer and the FDA agreed that if the list of side effects was too long, it would discourage people from taking the drug.[7]

GM: I'm always amazed by the TV commercials for drugs. They might be for restless leg syndrome or erectile dysfunction or something and they say, "May cause headaches, fatigue, nausea, diarrhea, dizziness, suicidal thoughts, stroke, heart failure, kidney failure, unusual bleeding, or sudden death." And I'm thinking, how badly do you want to keep your appendages in a certain position? I mean, after hearing these warnings, who the hell is buying these things?

PP: Well, the drug ads work because there are plenty of people out there who have these conditions. They go in and ask their doctor for the drugs, and the doctors feel as if they should accommodate their patients. What they should really do is say no. It's okay to say no to somebody. Of course, doctors worry that the patient will switch to the doctor down the street. My response would be to let them. Let them go to the doctor down the street and get the bad treatment. You don't get it here.

Even the way that adverse events are reported is manipulated by the drug companies and the FDA, in collusion with one another. You have an institutional conflict of interest with the FDA: the organization that approves drugs should not be regulating them in the marketplace. Why? Because in order to withdraw a drug, the FDA essentially has to admit that it was wrong to approve it. One step in the right direction, in addition to posting trials online in advance, would be requiring proof that the drug is not only better than nothing but also better than other drugs on the market. That way, we avoid the "me too" drugs that do no more than mimic other drugs. We should also split the FDA into two agencies—one that approves drugs and one that monitors safety. That way, the one that monitors safety in the marketplace might not be so inclined to allow a bad drug to stay on the market.

If you go back and look at the Merck debacle with Vioxx, you will find that for many, many years before that drug was taken off the market, the FDA knew, as did Merck, that the drug was seriously dangerous. The same thing is true for Accutane and Crestor. These are dangerous, terrible drugs; they shouldn't be taken by anybody. Yet the government didn't do anything about Vioxx until tens of thousands of people had died.[8]

The FDA is no less flawed when it comes to regulating supplements, functional foods, and fortified foods. The supplement and food industries have been able to influence decisions at the FDA for years. The FDA long ago succeeded, unintentionally, at getting public sentiment on the side of the supplement makers by using tactics that were so outrageous and over the top as to provoke a backlash. Before the Dietary Supplement Health and Education Act (DSHEA) of 1994 was passed, the FDA had done things like raid the office of a doctor who was making his own vitamin C formula. They used heavily armed Alcohol, Tobacco, Firearms and Explosives agents to hold people in the office at gunpoint as the agents confiscated the office records. That's an example of a kind of governmental overreach that breeds contempt of government. DSHEA got the FDA off the back of the supplement industry and allowed the supplement manufacturers to make generalized, unsubstantiated claims about how a given supplement may support the function of a given organ. The FDA is now toothless in dealing with the supplement industry, and given the history of the FDA, we're probably better off that way.

GM: The FDA may be ineffective when it comes to doing things like pulling dangerous drugs off the market, but it can be remarkably effective and tenacious opposing nonconventional forms of treatment.

PP: Oh exactly, exactly, because their real client is the drug companies. If you look at most of the decisions that the FDA makes, it's acting in the interest of the drug companies. When Andrew von Eschenbach was head of the FDA, Avastin was approved for breast cancer treatment. It does not extend the life of breast cancer patients by a single day, but signing that order resulted in billions of dollars in sales for Genentech.[9]

That decision benefited Genentech, but it did not benefit most of the women who took the drug. And while people love to beat up the insurance companies over these issues, consider the plight of an insurance company that was forced to pay $90,000—that's what Avastin costs the average patient annually—for a drug that does absolutely nothing at all, because the drug companies lobby Congress to force Medicare to pay for it. Once Medicare pays, then all the insurance companies have to pay. We like to beat up the insurance companies, but they're being mandated to pay for a lot of ineffective treatment, yet still have to make a profit, make their shareholders happy, and pay for all these unnecessary diagnostic tests and annual visits to the doctors and on and on and on. So the whole system is screwed up and the FDA is a vital cog in that very screwed-up wheel.

GM: Still, it's the USDA, not the FDA, that comes up with the Food Pyramid, or the Happy Plate, or whatever it calls its recommendations now.

PP: That's correct—and in conjunction with the Department of Health and Human Services.

GM: How did the USDA get involved in deciding what the healthiest diet should be? Why do we trust an agency that's supposed to deal with farm issues to tell us what to eat?

PP: We shouldn't. The conflict of interest stares us in the face. Its recommendations are all about promoting certain sectors of agriculture, not about what the healthiest diet should be. The most blatant example of the corruption is the "checkoff" program.

GM: Explain how that works.

PP: With the dairy checkoff, for example, for every hundred pounds of milk that dairy producers sell, they are mandated to contribute fifteen cents to the program. That money is spent on marketing dairy products to the public, like the "Got Milk?" campaign. It's also spent on direct marketing of dairy products to schools, on promoting the use of butter, on partnering with fast-food chains to offer more cheese in their pizzas or more milk in their coffees, and on research to create new and more devastating uses of dairy.

But it's not only dairy. There's also a pork and a beef checkoff program. Cattle producers pay a dollar a head. Let me read to you from a website funded by the beef checkoff program a little ditty called "Feel Good about Loving Beef":

> Isn't it great that a food you crave can be so good for you too? Beef is easy to love because it tastes so great, but it's also a naturally nutrient-rich source of ten essential nutrients. The protein in beef helps strengthen and sustain your body. Evidence shows that protein plays an important role in maintaining healthy weight, building muscle and fueling physical activity. And when you've got all that going for you, you and your loved ones are one big step closer to a healthier lifestyle and at lower risk for disease.[10]

GM: That's very nice. Conservatives are always saying that government should get out of the way and let private businesses run things efficiently without bureaucratic interference. But the checkoff program seems to me a good example of government and business working in complete harmony on a disinformation campaign.

PP: Yes. Working hand in hand to help make people sick and obese.

GM: Does the FDA get involved in nutrition at all?

PP: It gets involved only to the extent that it regulates, along with the Federal Trade Commission, the sale of supplements and the approval for structure/function claims that can be made about certain nutrients and the labeling of fortified functional foods. So we can thank the FDA, for example, for allowing cholesterol-lowering claims to be made for margarine products that are 100 percent fat because the companies fortify the margarine with beta sitosterol or plant sterols, which have been known to lower cholesterol.

GM: You're kidding me? In other words, you could take pork fat, inject a little bit of niacin in it, and make a cholesterol-lowering claim for that?

PP: Basically, yeah. You've come up with a viable business model.

GM: But it doesn't seem kosher.

PP: And this constant bantering back and forth that goes on between the FDA and the food companies about fortifying foods by adding omega-3s to white bread, and the health claims that can be made for that nonsense, is unconscionable. If we want to reduce the incidence of coronary artery disease, for example, that means that we've got to, on the federal level, start giving people the right advice. Here's why it's not happening. If you give the people the right advice, it means you're going to tell them to eat more of something, less of something, and none of something.

147

Then you're going to tick off manufacturers and agricultural groups, something the government is unwilling to do. So whose side is the government on? It's willing to sacrifice tens of millions of people to horrible treatments, drugs, unnecessary procedures, and even deaths every year so that it doesn't tick off the National Dairy Council? So that it doesn't upset Kellogg's? That's who the federal government is working for, not us. It does not function in the interest of the public health.

GM: Do you have a theory about whether the decision makers at the FDA—and for that matter the AND, the AMA, and so forth—believe that they're doing the right thing? Do you think that they're simply in the dark scientifically, but that they at least believe that the science is on their side? Or do you think that they know that what they're promoting is untrue and evil and corrupt, but they're just making a living?

PP: I think some of both. First of all, health care professionals in general often do not have a very good understanding of how to read and interpret research. A common issue is reporting data in relative versus absolute terms. For example, patients are told that a 50 percent reduction in the recurrence of breast cancer results from taking tamoxifen. And boy, with those results, who wouldn't take it, right? Then you discover the recurrence rate is 1.3 percent; with tamoxifen, recurrence is reduced to 0.68 percent, which is actually a 49 percent reduction, but the real or absolute benefit to the patient taking tamoxifen is one-half of 1 percent.[11] Once someone looks at the side effects, nobody in her right mind would say, "Oh, I'm willing to endure all of this to reduce my risk of a recurrence of breast cancer by half a percent; it's an insane trade-off." So, part of it is well intentioned but poor science, combined with a mind-set that all the solutions to our problems must be drug related. They view their findings through that filter.

And then the other side of it is just pure money. We're not going to tick off anybody who's in a position to hurt us. The late Senator George McGovern learned that lesson long ago, and it's had a chilling effect that's lasted decades.

GM: What happened to Senator McGovern?

PP: Senator McGovern chaired a Senate committee that started looking into a shift from Americans being malnourished to Americans suffering from diseases of excess. And he had Ancel Keys testify in front of his committee. Keys had done the Seven Countries Study that helped establish the role of cholesterol in cardiovascular disease. As a result, Senator McGovern and his committee issued some dietary recommendations; you and I wouldn't like them a whole lot, but they're a whole lot better than the guidelines at the time. They discouraged overreliance on animal foods and processed foods. The food business—the agriculture groups—were incensed by this and got together, determined to take him out. Senator McGovern lost his bid for re-election in large part because of the enormous amounts of money that came from the cattlemen's associations and the dairy industry and the agriculture groups that said this guy's bad for business. So all the politicians looked around and said, "You know what, it's not profitable to stand up to the agri-foods complex."

GM: In the end, the recommendations of the USDA and the FDA and the AND tend to get filtered through doctors, so let's talk about medical doctors. They get how many hours, typically, of training in nutrition?

PP: Tufts University is the best and those doctors get seventeen hours; that's not seventeen credit hours; that's seventeen class-room hours in nutrition. They're the best in the country.

GM: And the worst?

PP: That would be about three-fourths of them, where the subject's not even discussed at all. And in most of the rest, a cursory review of nutrition is about the best you can hope for. I've had current medical students tell me that when the subject of nutrition comes up, it's dismissed as inconsequential. Their attitude is that patients can always be referred to a dietitian or whatever. There is absolutely no awareness—and this is true for all health care professionals. Nobody is taught that diet is the cause of the diseases we battle and nobody is taught that diet will reverse them. A doctor or a dietitian or a nurse practitioner or a physician assistant who goes to school is not taught that you can reverse early-stage multiple sclerosis with diet. They're not taught that diet causes it and they're not taught to reverse it. In fact, none of them are taught to reverse any condition. They're taught to treat symptoms with drugs.

GM: Now, we can assume that most med school students are highly intelligent.

PP: Undoubtedly.

GM: Is it possible that they could go to med school for four years and, even if they're not taught anything about nutrition in med school, not see the relationship between, for example, diet and heart disease, and just focus on pharmaceutical and surgical interventions?

PP: Well, even if they see the relationship, they need to be quiet about it. Friends of mine who are physicians advocating a low-fat, plant-based diet in their medical practice have children who have applied to medical school and mentioned in their essays their interest in helping patients regain and maintain their health with diet. Their applications were met with disinterest and in sometimes open hostility; in one instance, an applicant was instructed to sanitize his application of this information in order to be considered.

GM: All the same, there are obviously many doctors who give advice about diet, even if they've had no formal training in the subject. I would think that most doctors who have patients with heart disease discuss with them whether hamburgers or cheeseburgers or hot dogs are a good idea. I mean, even the general public knows that cheeseburgers contribute to heart disease.

PP: There are a few things that need to be said about the advice that people do get from doctors. The first is that doctors tell patients to reduce the fat, lose a few pounds, to try to eat less red meat. They buy into the myth that if you eat chicken and fish instead of red meat, it will help you tame your coronary artery disease, which we know is not true. The second thing is that the recommendations tend to be so general that the person has no idea what to do with them. One thing that we've learned at The Wellness Forum is that the specificity of the instruction has a lot to do with the outcome. If I tell you, "Hey, Glen, eat a little bit less of this," you don't really know what that means. If I say, "Glen, do not eat this; I want you to eat that instead," you now have a specific directive. The likelihood that you'll know what to do and be able to follow through on all my advice is a much greater. The information from doctors tends to be vague; in the context of the short office visit, that's about as good as it's going to get. The third thing is that some doctors don't even do that much. They basically say, "Okay, you have coronary heart disease and high cholesterol, but your dad had it and your grandfather had it. It runs in families, so the earlier we treat you with meds or an angioplasty, the better."

The patient is effectively told that he or she is the helpless victim of bad genetic wiring. That victim mentality shines through and sometimes precludes any advice whatsoever about diet from being dispensed, or taken to heart if it is.

GM: There's also the problem of low expectations, isn't there? Doctors may recognize that meat and cheese in the diet are harmful, but believe that it's all but impossible for most people to change their eating habits.

PP: Yes, that's a problem. The idea that either people won't try it or they won't stick with it—that's taken as gospel, although there are some studies out there that suggest otherwise. You know, Dr. Neal Barnard did the original compliance study on Dr. Dean Ornish's diet and showed that patients who made bigger changes were more compliant and happier with their diets.[12] He conducted a similar study with diabetic patients who converted to a plant-based diet that showed similar results.[13]

GM: If doctors believe that their patients can't possibly change their diet and they approach them with that philosophy, then that's likely going to be self-reinforcing: patients will embrace what's presented as the difficulty of changing one's diet.

PP: The more insidious aspect is getting unhelpful dietary advice. Let's say I develop high cholesterol and high blood pressure and I go to a traditional doctor. Perhaps she is even enlightened enough to have a dietitian in the office. However, that dietitian is trained on the party line, so the dietitian says I've got to have skim milk on the cereal, give up hamburgers and cheeseburgers and pizza, but I can have some chicken and fish. So I really work at this, I'm trying. I'm drinking the skim milk that tastes like crap and eating a lot of salmon. I do this for six months and I show back up at my doctor's office. My cholesterol's actually gone up and my A1C levels, a marker for diabetes, have also gone up. I had a prediabetic condition and now it looks like it's developing into full-blown diabetes despite my best efforts for six months and you know what I say? "This dietary change doesn't work, give me the drugs." And so the medical skepticism about diet becomes a self-fulfilling prophecy because the dietary advice given out has no chance of helping anybody.

On the other hand, when we put people on the type of diet that actually does work, we get a different form of reinforcement. People get better, they lose weight, they get off their medications, and they don't want to go back. We get a great deal of compliance because they actually see results from their effort. And that's the big missing link in what's going on in the general medical community.

Doctors need to know, and I believe most of them do, that part of their job, if they're going to be in practice and present themselves as doing right by people, is to continue to learn. It's the responsibility of any physician in practice to be reading and learning all the time. Now, it would be lovely if one way they would continue their learning would be by visiting, say, Dr. McDougall's Health and Medical Center in Santa Rosa, California, or our Wellness Forum in Columbus, Ohio. But that's not what happens. Doctors go to continuing education conferences that are largely sponsored by drug companies. The companies have doctors make presentations about the use of their drugs, many of which are off-label applications, which the drug reps can't recommend, but doctors and continuing medical education programs effectively can.

GM: Now, doesn't a lot of that additional education sponsored by drug companies take place at resorts in places like Maui?

PP: Oh yeah, and on cruise ships. And you get to be a presenter by being a high prescriber. There are rewards for being a high

153

prescriber. For example, you and your spouse get an all-expenses-paid vacation for making a presentation on how to prescribe for off-label uses. So even the system of continuing education for doctors is corrupt.

GM: I didn't know about the rewards for being a high prescriber. I've never seen a doctor advertise on a website, "Number-one prescriber of Fosamax." Why is that?

PP: Professional modesty.

MANAGING
YOUR DOCTOR

. . . .

GM: Pam, what do you see as the ideal role of doctors in people's lives? Should people go for annual checkups? Should they do any tests to monitor their health?

PP: No. *Newsweek* had a cover story titled "One Word Can Save Your Life: No!"[1] It's about saying no to diagnostic tests. The article doesn't make quite as strong a statement as either I or Dr. John McDougall would, but it's right up there. It basically pointed out that the more tests you have, the more likely you are to discover something that's insignificant but get treatment for anyway. Most major organizations, including the U.S. Preventive Services Task Force, have said that there's no value to the annual exam.[2] One interesting point that Dr. McDougall makes when he speaks about this issue, and it had a profound effect on me, is that he grew up where you go to the doctor every year for a physical. He said during that time he gained fifty pounds, he developed an intestinal obstruction, had to have surgery, and had a stroke. Obviously, the annual physical did him no good at all. The annual exam, the way we've structured it, is absolutely useless, so I don't go. I don't think you'll find many people who are involved in this plant-foods movement spending much time in doctors' offices. Probably the further away you get from doctors, the better off you're going to be, in most cases.

GM: All right, let me play devil's advocate here. I've always gone for annual checkups. For many years, my cholesterol was about 160 or so and then it started creeping up. I told you the story about how, a little bit more than a year ago, it went as high as 212. That's when I spoke to Dr. McDougall. He told me to cut out the fructose; now I'm back down to my normal levels again. If I hadn't gone for an annual checkup, I wouldn't have known I was at 212. I would have thought, "Gee, I'm on a great diet. I'm fine." I would have continued eating my few cookies in the evening and my sweetened soy yogurt and so forth. I had a significant problem brewing and I learned about it only from my annual checkup.

PP: First of all, you're a little more enlightened than the average person, and have been for quite some time. Second, you didn't have a doctor, obviously, who was trying to get you to do more than just come in, check in, get a blood test, and go home. Third, you were lucky enough to be able to discuss your problem with Dr. McDougall.

You're not the one I'm concerned about, Glen. I'm concerned about the average healthy male who shows up and the doctor says, "Let's do a prostate-specific antigen (PSA) test because you're getting to that age where you ought to have one." So you get a

PSA test and it's a little bit elevated. Soon they identify a few cancer cells and you're rushed into having a prostatectomy. Now, in all likelihood, if you had done nothing, if you had never known about those funny cells, you would die with that cancer at the age of ninety-seven—die with it, but not of it.

I'm concerned about the woman who goes to the OB/GYN's office for her annual checkup, and the doc tells her she needs a mammogram. As a result, they discover a carcinoma in situ and next thing you know, she's labeled a cancer patient. She has surgery, she's taking tamoxifen, and she's had enough radiation to increase her risk of a heart disease significantly. Those are the more typical scenarios, which is why the whole situation is so inadvisable for people. What I tell people is, first of all, learn what the research shows in terms of results from common diagnostic tests. Once you do, you're likely to do none of this diagnostic testing that doctors want to subject you to, and I'm not talking about a blood test to get your cholesterol tested. My gosh, you can go to a drugstore and get that done now; you don't even need to go to see a doctor.

In my books and lectures, I advise people to do none of these diagnostic tests that you're being pushed to do when you go in, whether it's a Dexa scan, PSA, mammogram, colonoscopy, etc.; they're not going to save your life. All they do is lead to more tests and more treatments that don't work. A blood panel is fine only if you are a smart consumer about medicine. Here's what I mean by that. In your case, you go to the drugstore, get a blood test, see that your cholesterol is up—notice that you didn't ask your doctor what do to about it, you asked Dr. McDougall what to do. What do you think would have happened if the average person asked the doctor what to do about it?

GM: Probably a statin.

157

PP: Yeah. Because it runs in your family, Glen. That's the type of advice that you would get. So to be a smart medical consumer, you decide what steps to take on your own behalf. You may want to look for any way to do so outside of the traditional medical establishment.

Now, if I had a relentless pain in my side, I didn't know what it was, and it didn't go away by Monday, I would clearly go see a doctor. That's smart medical consumerism. But showing up in this perfectly healthy state that I am in to say, "Listen, I just want you to poke and prod and tell me that I'm okay after as much poking and prodding as you can get my insurance company to pay for," well, that's where the problem is.

GM: So you believe in going to doctors if you feel pain or if something unusual is going on?

PP: Of course. A woman in her thirties misses four menstrual periods in a row and she's not pregnant—I think she ought to check it out.

GM: At that point, do you do whatever tests the doctor orders? How do you manage this relationship with the doctor?

PP: You should ask a lot of questions, but don't consent to anything until you have a complete understanding of it. You go to the doctor and say, "Look, I've got this pain on my side and I can't figure out what it is." And she says, "Well, we need to do some imaging." Okay, well, what kind of imaging? She might say a CT scan, but if you investigate CT scans, you may decide that that's way too much radiation and that you'll probably be better off with an MRI. What you really want to do is gather information. If you don't know the answers to some of these questions, go home, do some research, and then decide what you're going to do. I'm not saying you should dillydally for another nine months—you may be on a fairly tight schedule of needing to figure out what's wrong—but you don't just do what you're told. Some doctors will test you to within an inch of your life. Again, the worst thing you can have if you walk into a doctor's office or a hospital is great insurance because they're going to use it.

GM: What if they find a tumor and say we need to operate immediately?

PP: The number of times that a condition is so life-threatening that we find out about it this afternoon and we need to have surgery tomorrow morning is such a tiny percentage that it isn't even worth talking about. You say, "Great, I'd like to have any images and any other information that you can give me so that I'm really clear on what's going on with me." Take notes and then say, "Thank you so much, I'm really glad we've gotten to the bottom of this. Please tell me what you think I ought to do and I'm going to take real careful notes here. By the way, please understand when you're telling me what you want me to do, I would like some outcomes and expectations in absolute rather than relative terms. I want you to tell me the straight story. I'm going to go check this out with some other people, get some other opinions from people who have different tools in their toolbox, and then I'm going to make up my mind about what to do." And that's when you get in touch with somebody like me or Dr. Ralph Moss or Dr. McDougall, get some other points of view, and then make your best decision about what you think is right for you to do. Don't get herded into some type of procedure without looking into it first.

GM: Okay. What if a woman has a Pap test and they find pre-cancerous cells on the cervix, dysplasia, and she's told she needs a LEEP Cone biopsy? Isn't that potentially a lifesaver?

PP: Well, yes, but there's also a good chance that the treatment she was getting from the OB/GYN caused it in the first place; that's what happened to me.

GM: Say that again? A chance that the treatment she was getting caused the dysplasia?

PP: Yes. First of all, birth control pills are carcinogens; they're full of hormones. We know that supplemental hormones are carcinogenic; a lot of women get these conditions by taking birth control pills.[3]

That's what happened to me when I got cervical dysplasia. What added to it was the terrible diet that I was eating at the time; this episode took place about five years before my conversion. I also got the human papillomavirus, which is a minor player in the whole thing. However, all of this could have been avoided if I had been eating the right diet and hadn't been taking those dreadful pills. Even after you're diagnosed with dysplasia, if you get off the pills, stop drinking so much alcohol and eating dairy products, and eat the right foods, that condition will right itself most of the time.

Since it's not immediately life-threatening, it's one of those conditions where it's worth it to go home, practice dietary excellence, do the right things, go back to the doctor in four months and have another Pap smear, and see if it's gone away before you do anything about it. Keep in mind that the LEEP Cone biopsy procedure requires a general anesthetic, something that's best to avoid whenever possible. So, in my case, not only did this doctor who did the LEEP Cone biopsy give me the birth control pills, which were a major part of why I developed the condition in the first place, but I stayed on the birth control pills because he didn't tell me to stop taking them. I went home and continued to eat cheese and drink alcohol and eat cookies for another several years. So my risk of recurrence was huge; I'm lucky it didn't happen to me.

GM: But wouldn't a woman in that situation who delays the procedure feel that she's taking a risk that it may spread if the diet doesn't control it?

PP: That's why you put a stop-loss on it. You don't walk out the door and say, "I'm just going to go change my diet and I'm never coming back here again." There are ways to figure out if it's progressing, staying the same, or regressing. If it's staying the same, you don't do anything about it because it can't kill you unless it progresses. Medicine does have a way of quantifying the situation. That's why it's so important to be knowledgeable. At The Wellness Forum, the information we provide about this type of topic is as important as how to eat the diet; if you don't understand how to manage your relationship with your doctor, you could be just as victimized by the health care profession and end up in just as much trouble.

You have to gain enough knowledge and confidence to go in and tell the doctor, "I hear what you're saying and I appreciate that because you have malpractice insurance and a medical license, you have to tell me certain things. Go ahead and note it in the file. I'll even sign something saying that you told me this stuff. But I've learned enough about this now, having looked into it on my own, to know that there's absolutely nothing to be lost by waiting three or four months to see if this condition clears up when I stop fertilizing it. I understand now that I've been fertilizing it with alcohol, cheese, sugar, and birth control pills. I'm going to try to protect myself now by eating a lot of whole foods, including lots that are rich in folate."

161

GM: I think we need to acknowledge that one reason for over-testing is the legitimate fear on the part of doctors of medical liability.

PP: Certainly true, but on the other hand I accompanied a friend to the ER with a sinus infection, and the doc recommended an MRI—for a sinus infection. I don't think he was worried about being sued. Consumers should be especially wary of doctors who do tests inside their own offices, because they have the strongest financial incentive to overtest, but the root of the problem is deeper than just greed.

GM: Let's review different types of testing and get your opinion about the harmful effects, if any, of each type. I know that you're an opponent of mammograms. Is there ever a use for mammograms, or are they always worthless?

PP: I would never agree to one myself. I think they're worthless.

GM: I would imagine that this is fairly shocking to most women who have all been told that mammography can and does save lives.

PP: Remember, though, that these are marketing messages for mammography, not messages reporting the scientific findings.

Mammography is highly unreliable. It tends to miss aggressive tumors that grow between screenings, while detecting small, benign tumors, such as carcinoma in situ, that are usually not cancers at all and are often referred to as "pseudo-cancers." As a reminder, the word "pseudo" means "false." It's a false cancer.

In spite of the fact that most of these pseudo-cancers will not develop into a cancer that will require treatment, women diagnosed with them are advised to have lumpectomies, to receive radiation treatments, and to take drugs like tamoxifen. This is overtreatment for a condition that is highly unlikely to be life-threatening. Particularly troubling is how these women are classified as "cancer survivors." Almost all of them would be alive five years after diagnosis (the benchmark for survival for cancer patients) even with no treatment. This skews the survival statistics numbers, making it look like treatments for breast cancer are much more effective than they really are.

While mammography detects pseudo-cancers resulting in overtreatment, it does not reduce the risk of dying from real cases of breast cancer.

A research letter published in 2001 in *Lancet* reported the findings of a Cochrane Review that looked at the efficacy of mammograms for reducing breast cancer deaths. It is important to note that the Cochrane Collaboration is the most independent medical research organization in the world, and therefore its conclusions about various issues related to medicine are taken more seriously by many of us.

The article stated, "In 2000, we reported that there is no reliable evidence that screening for breast cancer reduces mortality. As we discuss here, a Cochrane Review has now confirmed and strengthened our previous findings."[4]

Cochrane has further concluded that screening led to an increase in radical treatments due to overdiagnosis of 25 to 35 percent; that 49 percent of screened women would experience at least one false positive; and that the absolute reduction in risk of death was 0.1 percent.[5]

The Cochrane researchers also concluded that studies showing that mammograms reduce the risk of dying from breast cancer do not take into consideration the deaths related to breast cancer treatments, and that more women are harmed from overtreatment than are saved with mammography. The groups stated, "There is no reliable evidence from large randomized trials to support screening mammography at any age."

163

Another study published online by the *British Medical Journal*[6] was conducted in Denmark, a great country for studying mammography outcomes. For the past seventeen years, only about 20 percent of women in Denmark have been screened, leaving a large control group from which data can be gathered.

Two geographic areas were included in the study: Copenhagen, where screening was introduced in 1991; and Funen, where screening was introduced in 1997. Between 1997 and 2005, deaths from breast cancer dropped by 5 percent for women between the ages of thirty-five and fifty-five in both of these areas. For women between fifty-five and seventy-four, the decline was 1 percent in mortality rate.

In the nonscreened population in Denmark, the death rate from breast cancer declined by 6 percent for women between the ages of thirty-five and fifty-five, and 2 percent for women between fifty-five and seventy-four.

The researchers also observed that the diagnosis of carcinoma in situ doubled in the population of women who were screened and remained the same in the nonscreened population, reinforcing the idea that mammography results in overdiagnosis of pseudo-cancers.

Studies even show that mammography is contraindicated for women who carry the BRCA1 or BRCA2 gene mutation, which predisposes them to a higher risk of developing breast cancer. In one study, researchers concluded that mammography screening beginning at twenty-five to twenty-nine years of age results in a higher risk of breast cancer due to increased lifetime radiation exposure, and that mammography may have a net harmful effect for these patients.[7]

GM: What do you say to the person who reports that a friend or family member was diagnosed with breast cancer via mammography and it saved her life?

PP: Since the data is clear that more women are harmed than helped, this is highly unlikely. In other words, what has happened in most cases, where women truly have survived and thrived for a long time, is that they were diagnosed with pseudo-cancer and treated for it. The treatments for metastasized breast cancer are not much more effective today than they were decades ago.

Another thing I would add is that, according to Cochrane, if two thousand women are screened for ten years, one woman will benefit from early detection. You may happen to know the one in two thousand who actually benefitted, but it's statistically unlikely.

One of the best resources for understanding this issue is Peter Gotzsche's book *Mammography Screening: Truth, Lies and Controversy*. It's a technical book, but I would love to see it become required reading for women since this is such an important issue.

GM: Let's move on to CT scans.

PP: In certain situations they can be valuable, but because the dose of radiation is so high, and it's a well-established fact that CT scans increase your risk of cancer,[8] they really should be reserved for situations where it's the only way to get the information you need. They're way overused.

GM: And they're highly overused with children, isn't that right?

PP: Yes. Not only are they overused but they're overused on the same people—individuals getting multiple scans. It's not unusual to see CT scans that make the whole situation so much worse for them. CT scans should be the last resort, not the first line of action; unfortunately that's not the way it goes.

GM: MRIs?

165

PP: Valuable and less dangerous. For example, in the case of breast cancer, it can sometimes be a valuable way to find out exactly what's going on. The biggest risk may be that because the imaging is so good, you're going to discover something else that you don't want to know about. I was at a dinner party last night and listened to the story of a woman who is one of those people who goes to doctors all the time. She's overmedicated and doesn't want to hear what I have to say, so I just listened.

She apparently got an MRI for one reason, but they found something in her brain that they weren't looking for. They sent her to specialists; she went through ninety days of testing and was scared half to death. The specialists put her on Coumadin because they weren't sure it wasn't a blood clot, but then found out that there was some type of tangled or turned vein in her brain. If you spend too much time allowing doctors to poke and prod you, you're liable to find out things that you're better off not knowing. The last doctor she saw about her condition said, "This isn't even worth spending time on. Go live your life and forget about it." Which was good advice, but that's after ninety days, $10,000 worth of tests, and thinking she either had a brain tumor or was going to drop dead any minute. That's a pretty frightening situation to be in for nothing at all.

GM: Ultrasounds?

PP: Not dangerous and very helpful sometimes. These are the least invasive of all of the forms of testing.

GM: There's really no risk to doing an ultrasound, right?

PP: The main risk, and this is true of all forms of imaging, is finding something you may not want to know about.

GM: Would you say the same thing about ultrasounds for pregnant women?

PP: Today, having an ultrasound is a routine part of medical care for pregnant women. No one questions it, but the problem is that it often finds things that look suspicious, even when there is nothing wrong. One analysis of fifty-six studies showed that follow-up testing for abnormalities detected as a result of ultrasound would result in more miscarriages than confirmed diagnoses.[9]

GM: So ultrasounds aren't inherently bad, but it sounds like they cause more problems than they prevent sometimes. What about other imaging procedures?

PP: There is a great book on this topic by Dr. Gilbert Welch called *Overdiagnosed.* I recommend that all of our members read it. It describes how imaging and testing tends to identify clinically insignificant abnormalities that would be better left alone, but this is seldom the response to finding them. Tiny abdominal aneurisms and small thyroid nodules are examples of conditions often found in completely asymptomatic people who are subjected to testing. All imaging, including ultrasounds, should be used with caution. In the book, Dr. Welch[10] discusses the new epidemic of thyroid cancer. How did we suddenly get an epidemic of thyroid cancer? Is it something in the water? No, what's happening is that people are getting X-rays and MRIs and they're finding thyroid cancer. They're not necessarily looking for it, but they end up with an image of it, anyway. A lot of people have little nodules on their thyroids, which they now call cancer. They are then advised to have to have surgery for it because the American Cancer Society has gone all out to make sure everybody now gets screened for the new epidemic of thyroid cancer!

GM: Well, I have a friend who it happened to. He had an ultrasound performed for neck pain, and they found a nodule on his thyroid, completely unrelated to the pain, of course. They did a biopsy and told him he has cancer. He faces the choice of an operation with serious risks or "watchful waiting." I'm certain he'll opt for the "watchful waiting." I asked him if he would rather never have known. He didn't hesitate for a moment. He would much rather never have known. The diagnosis has taken an enormous emotional toll on him and his family, to no good end.

Let's move on to another test. Is there any point to an angiogram?

PP: The value of it really would be to scare somebody half to death. To put the image up there, if doctors did this right, and say, "See this? This is going to kill you. Now, medicine says I'm supposed to put a stent in that artery. I can do it, I know how to do it, I'm trained to do it; I'm just telling you it's useless, even though your insurance company will pay for it. Or you can change your diet. If you don't change your diet, this is going to kill you." So it has some value in terms of scaring people a little bit, if doctors would be willing to engage in the right conversation with their patients. Unfortunately, that's not what they're doing.

GM: Okay, if somebody was having chest pain and was willing and eager to start a change of diet and lifestyle that you would endorse, would there be any point in his doing an angiogram? Or should he just get started eating a low-fat, plant-based diet?

PP: He should just start eating the low-fat, plant-based diet. Now, there are factors like how much chest pain, was there a myocardial infarction, have there been previous events? It's hard to answer these questions in general because, in the real world, they're always specific, which is why people really should consult with a medical doctor. But if your current doctor won't discuss the importance of diet and won't even entertain the idea that you ate your way into coronary artery disease and will probably be able to eat your way out of it, you may want to consider finding another doctor. There are docs who are more open-minded, even if they don't completely understand the issues we've been discussing.

GM: Are there any times you feel a situation is so severe that, even though they're going to eat their way out of it, it might help them now to have either a surgical intervention or a pharmaceutical intervention?

PP: Yes. If there is severe damage to the left ventricle, I'd think we'd all agree, then bypass surgery is probably valuable then. The other is relentless chest pain, which is not usually the way these patients present. They usually present with intermittent chest pain or pain from exertion. But if somebody has constant, relentless chest pain and it keeps him from sleeping, I think that person should be in the care of a good interventional cardiologist because surgery is needed. I would endorse it under that scenario.

There are few drugs or surgeries that I would say have absolutely no value. It's the misapplication of them that causes me to say the things that I do. I don't think we should eliminate bypass surgery. I'm saying instead of performing five hundred thousand of them annually, we should perform about fifteen thousand.

GM: What about colonoscopies? During my first checkup after I turned fifty, my rather humble and very decent doctor said to me, "You know, Glen, honestly, there isn't a lot that doctors can do for people, but the colonoscopy is one thing we do that's really helpful for the general public. I recommend having one at fifty." And I said, "Well, are there any downside risks?" He said, "Occasionally, we perforate the colon." I said, "Hey, it's been very nice visiting with you, doc."

PP: They've now found out that the colonoscopy is not any more valuable than a sigmoidoscopy. A couple of researchers at Columbia University looked at three different studies and determined that a colonoscopy does not offer any advantages over a sigmoidoscopy.[11] However, it does offer significantly more risk, and the pleasure of a tube up your rectum, if that's something you've always pined for.

GM: Exactly what is a sigmoidoscopy?

PP: Sigmoidoscopy involves the use of a flexible endoscope. It provides a view of the large intestine from the rectum to the sigmoid, the most distal part of the colon. It does not allow examination of the entire bowel, but the portion that is examined is where colorectal cancer is most likely to occur.

GM: So should people do a sigmoidoscopy?

PP: I wouldn't have one. By eating a high-fiber, low-fat diet, people will reduce their risk of colon cancer as much as they possibly can.

GM: What's the value of a PSA test, in your opinion?

PP: Zero. Worthless. And that's not just my opinion, that's also the opinion of Dr. Richard Ablin, who discovered the PSA protein. To his credit, he's said that he didn't realize that his discovery would lead to "the overdiagnosis, the overtreatment, and the billions of dollars that are basically wasted on a test that can't do what it's purported to do."[12]

Furthermore, the U.S. Preventive Services Task Force has now said that PSA tests are useless and men should not have them. The task force's conclusions were based on five clinical trials that showed PSA testing does not save lives and that having the test leads to more tests and treatments that cause impotence, incontinence, and other side effects.[13]

The lead researcher, Dr. Virginia Moyer, stated, "Unfortunately, the evidence now shows that this test does not save lives. This test cannot tell the difference between cancers that will and will not affect a man during his natural lifetime. We need to find one that does."

GM: And the Dexa scan for osteoporosis is worthless?

PP: Completely.

GM: How about genetic testing to find out if you have the genes for breast cancer or something?

PP: Harmful, terrible. It labels people as patients. It turns them into victims.

GM: The case for genetic testing is that it simply makes people aware of their risk profile.

PP: Yeah, and then you have to live with that information.

I had a member who recovered from an autoimmune disease who's doing quite well, actually. She has been practicing dietary excellence. Her sister died of ovarian cancer, so her family and her doctor pressured her to undergo genetic testing. They found that she had the gene mutation that predisposed her to have ovarian cancer, so the doctor removed her ovaries. While taking them out, they found out that she had some diverticular pouches, so they recommended a colonoscopy.

She asked me for my opinion. I said, "I want you to think about what's happened in the last thirty days. You were happy, living your life with two ovaries; now you've had two ovaries removed

171

and the doctor wants to do a colonoscopy. When are you going to stop this? How much more are you going to let them do to you? You have two well-formed bowel movements every day; you have no bowel problems. Those diverticular pouches are probably left from the days when you were a cheese eater."

If these interventions just stopped with notifying someone she is carrying the gene mutation and she could put it in the back of her head and forget about it, that would be great. But *nobody* puts it in the back of her head and forgets about it. We think we have to do something about it. Human beings are designed and engineered to solve problems; generally speaking, that's a pretty good idea. If I have a flat tire, I need to get a new tire; we've got to solve that problem. But when you get into a lot of these tests with their dubious results about genetic predispositions, all you're doing is putting terrible stress on people who are not medically knowledgeable. You may be solving a problem you don't have.

GM: What about Pap tests?

PP: While I don't oppose the Pap test as much as the others, its importance has been overstated, and the test too often results in overtreatment. According to Dr. Welch in *Overdiagnosed*, a fifteen-year-old girl who has annual Pap tests has a 75 percent chance of eventually having a colposcopy[14] (the procedure to biopsy abnormal cells). There is no watchful waiting or dietary change recommended in response to an abnormal Pap, and the treatments range from simple freezing with local anesthesia in the doctor's office to hysterectomy. The American College of Obstetrics and Gynecology now recommends that screenings start much later and be performed less frequently.[15]

172

GM: I wonder if the tide is turning. Nine medical societies, taking part in an initiative of a group called Choosing Wisely, have come up with a list of forty-five dubious medical services, most involving testing.[16, 17]

PP: That's a long overdue first step.

GM: Let's turn to mental health. Can diet be related to the condition of depression?

PP: It can be. First, there are a lot of people being diagnosed with depression who are eating a terrible diet; they're dehydrated, sedentary, out of shape, tired, have no energy, have low sex drives, sleep poorly, and suffer other related symptoms. These are also common symptoms of depression. I think some doctors are quick to label patients as depressed when there are other things going on. Sometimes an optimal diet, drinking adequate water every day, and exercise will cause the person to feel better, to have more energy, feel more clearheaded, sleep better, have an improved sex drive, and other noticeable improvements.

Then we have people who are depressed for visible reasons, such as the loss of a loved one or a job. We are labeling everyday stress and disappointment as depression and medicating people for it, when what they really need is just time to process their emotions.

Even for those who are truly clinically depressed, diet is important; they will feel better and think better, which will help them to get more out of therapy and to resolve their problems. Of course, nobody is saying that diet is the whole remedy; a truly depressed person won't overcome his issues with broccoli.

For the clinically depressed, therapy can be helpful if it is the right type of therapy. I recommend Cognitive Behavioral Therapy (CBT), which has been shown to be very effective for treating conditions like depression, anxiety, ADHD, and other mental and emotional disorders. It works quickly—usually fourteen sessions or so—there's a very low recidivism rate, and drugs are rarely used. The therapists who practice CBT are to the mind and emotions what Dr. Caldwell Esselstyn and Dr. McDougall are to the cardiovascular system and the endocrine system.

If you seek help for depression, I think the first thing you should say to your doctor is that you're not interested in a pharmaceutical solution to your problem. You're interested in talking and working your way through it. Psychotropic drugs are being dispensed like candy in this country and their side effects, including addiction, can be highly destructive. You want to avoid them at all costs.

GM: What do you think underlies the overprescription of antidepressants?

PP: There's a real arrogance today to the practice of psychiatry. Right now, we know that taking antidepressant and antianxiety drugs not only increases your risk of suicide but they ultimately make people more depressed.[18] That's why people have to take multiple drugs, which have to be constantly switched out to be effective. Forty percent of the time, there's absolutely no response to the drugs at all,[19] other than the depression getting worse. However, it doesn't stop psychiatrists from prescribing them. The trend in the psychiatric profession is to do less and less talk therapy, so the profession is now attracting people who don't like people. They have no interest in relating to people; they don't want to talk to them, and they don't have to talk to them; they just prescribe drugs.

Doctors are very smart people, but I think many times we're admitting the wrong people to medical school. We're bringing people into the profession who are very bright and technically very proficient, but they don't have the right idea about what medical practice should be about: preventing, stopping, and reversing disease. So they go to work every day and get used to the idea that everybody gets worse, everybody has to have more drugs, everybody has to have more procedures. Most of them are still making a lot of money and don't really have much interest in changing anything. I suspect that many of them like remaining ignorant. When confronted with evidence, they'll get upset about being confronted, but many will just continue to do what they're doing.

GM: You know, you're remarkably antidrug and antisupplement for a woman named "Popper."

PP: Maybe I overcompensate.

GM: Out of curiosity, when was the last time you went to a medical doctor, Pam?

PP: That was in 1994, about nineteen years ago. A cat bit me, and I got an infection. I went to a doctor, told him I needed an antibiotic and which one I wanted, and got out of there in ten minutes.

I want to make it clear that I have nothing against doctors. I'll go back promptly the next time I need one.

PROVING THE CASE

....

GM: Before we discuss specific clinical evidence, let's talk about the fact that people are understandably confused by studies. You hear on the news that vitamin E is good for the heart and then you hear that vitamin E isn't good for the heart. Or you hear that fish oil lowers cholesterol and heart attacks and then you hear that it doesn't. Why do we get contradictory results? Can we believe any of these studies?

PP: The first thing that I tell everybody when I'm giving public lectures, or when they join The Wellness Forum, is that you should always look at every study with some skepticism. No study by itself is really important; it's a study taken into consideration with the preponderance of the evidence that either adds weight to its importance or completely discounts it altogether. For example, the dairy industry put out a study—yes, it actually did commission such a study—that showed that dairy helps people lose weight. So you read the headlines and you think, "Gosh, I'd better go get some ice cream and cheese to slim down." But if you look at all of the studies that have been done on the topic, and there are a couple dozen of them, only a couple show that dairy helps you lose weight. And, oh, by the way, they were done by the same guy at the University of Tennessee who was paid $1.7 million by the dairy industry for those studies. On top of which, it's patently illogical that calorie-rich, dense, fatty foods should help anyone lose weight.

And so when we take a look at all of the rest of what's out there, the preponderance of the evidence says these two studies are irrelevant. Then let's take an opposite example. Dr. Caldwell Esselstyn's study shows that you can reverse heart disease, stop its progression, and actually reverse it with diet. That alone is provocative, but then you add in the China Study, you look at all the population studies that show that people who eat more of a plant-centered diet have less heart disease, and you add in the rest of what we know, suddenly that one study with eighteen patients starts to seem significantly more important. I tell people not to get carried away with the latest study or the latest headline, but to take a deeper look and use their brains when they read something that sounds too good to be true.

There are also ways, which we expound upon in one of the classes we offer from time to time, to sort through nutritional confusion with research. We show people how to evaluate research and go through why they don't need to be concerned with short-term changes and biomarkers that may not be significant for their long-term health. Remember, we live in a country where people are dying with excellent blood work, so we need to weigh more heavily studies of health practices that produce improved quality of life and longevity than studies of health practices or drugs that produce better biomarkers. There are some guidelines that you can use to look at research even as a layperson and make some pretty good decisions about what's reliable and what's not reliable evidence.

GM: How did the researcher manage to devise two studies that showed dairy helps you lose weight? How did he rig the results?

PP: Well, you can do a lot of things. You can do some things with selection criteria. For example, if you wanted to skew a study to show that people eating a plant-based diet don't fare better than people eating meat, just make the selection criteria the answer to the question "Do you eat meat and dairy?" No other criteria involved. So you could choose to enroll in the study a 475-pound person (like Del used to be) who would say, "I'm vegan; no meat, no dairy, no fish." Obviously, he's doing something wrong or he wouldn't weight 475 pounds, so he's probably going to be worse off than the meat eaters. You then publish a study that states a plant-based diet isn't very helpful.

One thing that the drug companies do is recruit what we call "perfect patients." Let's say they need to find 1,700 people out of the more than three hundred million in our population to do a study on a new cholesterol lowering drug. Since they want to minimize the side effects, they find 1,700 people who have high cholesterol diagnosed for the first time recently and have absolutely nothing else wrong with them. The researchers put these perfect patients on the drug; their cholesterol goes down with minimal side effects. Once the drug gets approved, that's not how the general public will use it. The drug gets used by many people who are taking four or five other drugs and have lots of other things wrong with them, including side effects that are significantly more severe.

Another problem with studies is that the research can just be plain sloppy. I hate to say that, but in this day and age, particularly if there's industry funding, the study design is not carefully scrutinized. And universities, in my opinion, are simply happy to see money coming in. A lot of these researchers have to fund their own departments or offices, so the lure of money to produce a study that shows a certain result can really lead to some sloppy study design. They can also skew the interpretation of the results; the study may not actually isolate dairy as a causative factor in weight loss, or the results can be so vague or insignificant as to not make any difference, but it can be reported in relative terms as if it's significant.

And then the study may only see a two-pound difference in weight loss between two groups but it is reported as people who eat dairy products lost 50 percent more weight than the other group. Well, the first group lost four pounds and the second group lost six pounds, which is 50 percent more, but it's a pretty meaningless number. There are all kinds of things that researchers can do, ranging from selection criteria for the subjects to how they define and measure the outcome and at what intervals to measure it, to how they report the findings, whether they are framed in absolute or in relative terms.

Sometimes, too, you can portray an apparently positive outcome without taking the negative consequences into consideration. The obvious example in the diet business is the Atkins Diet. People lose weight on the Atkins Diet, but they also get sick. I've always said if the only thing we're considering is that "it works," then let's throw in everything that works. Cocaine addiction works for weight loss. I've had lots of cocaine addicts in this office over the years and they were all skinny people. Now, we can all agree that cocaine addiction would be a ridiculous approach to weight loss. Well, so is the Atkins Diet in terms of adverse health effects.

180   **GM:** There's also the matter, when an isolated food or diet is being studied, of what kind of diet it's being compared to. Very rarely

are studies, let's say of dairy or fish consumption, compared to a low-fat, plant-based diet; it's always compared to the standard American diet.

PP: Yeah, that's a big issue. And even when they do use a control group that is eating a plant-based diet, or they consider that the intervention diet, it's not a well-structured diet. Our chef ate his way to 475 pounds on a plant-based diet. Just giving up meat doesn't make you a healthy eater at all; it has to go beyond that. That's where the comparison group can make all the difference in the world in terms of showing a result.

Take Loren Cordain, the guy who promotes the Paleo Diet. One of the reasons his diet looks so good when he tells stories (and he doesn't use a lot of research—he tells a lot of stories) is that he takes people who are eating the standard American diet, which includes fast food and cheese and pizza and toaster pastries and all this stuff you shouldn't eat, and puts them on the Paleo Diet, which is heavy on meat, vegetables, and fruit. And they generally get better, since they've cut out dairy, refined sugars, and a lot of processed foods. So you conclude, "My gosh, the Paleo Diet is spectacular." Well, the Paleo Diet is spectacular compared to where people were before, but in terms of comparing it to people eating the diet that I recommend, it's not spectacular at all. What the comparison group is doing helps determine the value of these studies.

GM: I once called the lead researcher of a study that had led the national news; the study was that high profile. This was a 2002 study published in the *Journal of the American Medical Association* that found that dairy consumption reduces insulin resistance syndrome.[1] I found that very remarkable news, the idea that dairy could reduce insulin resistance and therefore reduce diabetes. Here's how the lead scientist designed the study: it was a self-reporting study; he divided foods people ate into three categories: dairy, non-dairy, and mixed. He didn't include data from the mixed group in his study because, well, I guess he found mixed foods inherently ambiguous. It turns out that cheeseburgers were considered mixed. Macaroni and cheese was mixed, and so were double-cheese pizzas; none of that was considered dairy. I mean, if a double-cheese pizza was mixed, I wondered, then what was considered pure dairy?

PP: Maybe deep-fried butter on a stick?

GM: Yeah, maybe deep-fried butter on a stick, although the sugary glaze could make it a mixed dish. You know, these are the kind of questions that only a highly trained scientist can answer. There are clearly some nuanced distinctions here that are over my head. But I'm pretty sure that if you suckled directly from the teat of a bovine, it was considered dairy.

I called the man up and said, "Look, you're claiming with evidence that excludes pizza and many other cheesy foods that insulin resistance can be reduced with dairy. Since you want to isolate the effect of dairy on insulin resistance, why don't you actually do a study that compares people who eat dairy in all its forms, including pizza, with people who eat no dairy at all and look at the results there?" And he said, "Hmm, that's an interesting idea." Like it took remarkable insight to come up with that. But I don't believe he's ever done that study.

PP: Because it's something that the dairy industry would never fund.

GM: In fact, I believe his study had been funded in part by General Mills. Okay, let's talk about some studies that you feel do have value.

PP: Well, let's start with the work of Dr. Esselstyn that I alluded to earlier. I want to start with him because his work has rightly garnered so much attention, leading Bill Clinton to essentially adopt the diet we recommend. What I like about Dr. Esselstyn's results is that they're based on clinical practice; they're clear, impossible to dispute, and really unimpeachable.

Back in the mid-1980s, Dr. Esselstyn took twenty-four cardiac patients and asked them to follow a low-fat vegan diet. The rules of his diet were simple: no animal foods, no oil, no refined grains, and no nuts. He did not ask his patients to eliminate alcohol. About 9 to 12 percent of the calories in the diet were from fat. It turned out that eighteen of the twenty-four patients were compliant with the diet. Those eighteen very sick individuals, some of whom had been all but given up for dead by standard medical practitioners, had collectively experienced forty-nine cardiovascular events in the eight years before they adopted Dr. Esselstyn's diet regimen. There had been four heart attacks, three strokes, seven bypass surgeries, and nine of the patients suffered from increasing angina attacks.

After dietary intervention, the blood cholesterol of the compliant patients had dropped from an average of 246 mg/dl to an average of 137 mg/dl.[2] Follow-up angiograms determined that not only had the progression of disease been reversed in all patients but at least eight had actually reversed their disease, meaning that there was a significant opening of their coronary arteries. With the exception of one participant who stopped being compliant with the diet six years into the program, there were no new cardiac events in any of the patients during the first twelve years of the program.

Now consider the odds. What are the chances that Dr. Esselstyn just got lucky and his eighteen patients by random chance happened to get healthy and avoid cardiac events for the twelve years on his diet after they had collectively suffered forty-nine of them in the prior eight years? For any single individual who had had several cardiac events in the prior eight years, you might estimate his chances as being one in ten that he'd manage to survive the next twelve years without another such event. For that to happen to all eighteen individuals based on random chance, you'd be looking at odds of one in 10 to the 18th power.

The efficacy of the diet becomes clearer still when you compare the results of those eighteen compliant patients with the six who dropped out of the study in the first year or so and went back to their old ways of eating. What happened to them was just what you'd expect. Reviewed by Dr. Esselstyn in 1998, their cases of heart disease all progressed, and they had four more bypass operations, increasing angina, heart failure, and one death. So it's just not possible to make the case that it could have been anything other than diet that was responsible for the remarkable results that Dr. Esselstyn achieved. It's also worth noting that Dr. Dean Ornish has conducted similar studies, with a slightly different but similarly low-fat diet, and more emphasis on lifestyle, and achieved comparable results. As Dr. Ornish once said about the question of evaluating studies, "The more significant the degree of change, the more likely it is that the change is not due to chance."[3] Well, the degrees of change in health outcomes that both Dr. Esselstyn and Dr. Ornish have achieved in clinical studies have been highly significant and parallel.

GM: So the efficacy of diet has been proven, but do we have studies to determine how important a role genes play?

PP: Yes. Many studies have demonstrated that genes are less important than diet. This is an important idea to communicate because many people have a very defeatist attitude about their health that gets reinforced by their very learned cardiologists and other medical doctors who say, "Well, it's certainly not surprising that you've developed diabetes. I've been treating your mother for diabetes for the last fifteen years and your grandfather died of it. Of course this was destined to happen to you, and because you're a helpless victim of this relentless disease, we have to put you on these medications."

It's often one of the reasons why people won't seek care from somebody else or get a second opinion; they just think they're stuck with it. I see this when people come to dinners here at The Wellness Forum. They'll come as a guest with somebody else; they really don't know much about what we do and they're just flabbergasted to find out. They'll raise their hands and say, "I have high cholesterol and I've done the diet thing; I've tried everything and I just can't get my numbers down. I've been taking statin drugs and my doctor says that's just the way it's going to be. Now you're telling me that you can get rid of that problem?" When I estimate a 95 percent chance that proper diet will rid them of that problem, they almost cannot believe it. It's breathtaking to them.

It's very important that people understand the difference between having a gene and genetic expression, and the effect that your behavior has on the expression of certain genes, including those that predispose you to developing diseases. We have lots of evidence.

First, we have migration studies that have shown that when people move from one area to another and start eating the typical diet of their new home, they soon have the same disease risk of the area to which they moved.[4] For example, Japanese women in the United States are significantly more likely to develop breast cancer than Japanese women living in Japan and other Asian countries.[5] One of the reasons is that the traditional Japanese diet is lower in fat, particularly saturated animal fat, than the typical Western diet. In the 1940s, breast cancer was relatively rare in Japan; at that time, the Japanese diet was comprised of less than 10 percent of calories from fat.[6] But within a short time after

185

moving to the United States, Japanese women have the same risk of breast cancer as American women.

Their genetic makeup does not change as they fly across the ocean to their new homes; the main cause is the increase in consumption of fat, particularly fat in animal foods. Their behavior changes when they get here—that's the cause of their health deterioration. One of the first such studies was published in the *Journal of the National Cancer Institute* in 1968; it demonstrated that when people migrate from one area to another and adopt the typical diet in their new home, they acquire the disease risk of the area to which they migrated.[7]

There are some interesting population comparisons that have been done. One of them involves the Pima Indians, who are essentially divided into two groups: one leads a mostly Westernized lifestyle in Arizona, consuming a diet high in animal protein and fat; the other eats a more traditional Indian diet in Mexico: a grain and starch-based diet, with potatoes, corn, rice, beans, and locally grown vegetables and fruit—a diet with more than fifty grams of fiber per day. So they have the same ethnicity, essentially the same genetic makeup, and are close geographically, yet we find a huge difference in the diabetes rates between one group and the other. Naturally, the far worse outcomes are with the Western diet and lifestyle habits.

GM: How big is the difference?

PP: Diabetes rates are about 38 percent in the Arizona Pima and 6.9 percent in the Mexican Pima, according to the 2006 study published in *Diabetes Care*.[8] That's a big difference for people who are essentially ethnically identical.

We have to educate people quite a bit to get this point across. I'll tell you an area where it affects public policy. This way of thinking is going to take a long time to shift, but controversy arises when insurance companies and other companies seek to reward people for improving their health and losing weight. There are always those who object that companies are discriminating when they reward people for improving their health, since they see people as helpless victims of their genetic history. If we assume that people have no control over their own health, it seems unfair to reward those who lose weight. How then do we compensate the people that can't possibly lose weight because everybody in their family's overweight? Well, this is the defeatist prevailing wisdom out there. We need to tell employers that for the very tiny percentage of employees who actually can't change their health status, then we agree—they shouldn't be penalized. But for the rest of the group who can do something about it, they should be rewarded for doing it and penalized if they don't. That's an area where this misconception about genetic predisposition really influences what can be done in the public arena.

GM: Let's move on to supplements, since a lot of studies are designed to demonstrate whether or not they provide a benefit.

PP: What we find is that the weight of the evidence shows over and over again that supplements fail to prevent, stop, or reverse any disease. Sometimes they're even harmful. The advocates of the supplements are not usually the conventional doctors, but rather complementary and alternative and integrative practitioners, who I refer to as "holistic pharmacists." They are gaining more traction every day because of dissatisfaction with the traditional medical community. That dissatisfaction is widespread, and I firmly understand its roots. But the holistic pharmacists say to treat your health problems with health supplements instead of drugs because they're natural and don't have the same toxic side effects.

The reality remains that treating symptoms instead of the underlying cause is a bad idea. You could argue that some of the

187

supplements are less toxic than the drugs, but they still don't solve the problem. You've just got a different method of symptom control. Second, it's premised on the same defeatism toward diet that conventional medicine offers: people won't eat the right diet, so we have to give them supplements. I totally disagree with that whole line of thinking. And if you look at the studies, they clearly show that you cannot make up for your dietary indiscretions by popping a couple of vitamin pills in the morning. Much of the public has bought into the attitude toward supplements that they're harmless. Even if they don't help you, they believe, supplements aren't toxic; the worst-case scenario is that you end up with expensive urine. I still hear a lot of comments like that.

In fact, there was a huge study reported in the *British Medical Journal* in 2006 that looked at tens of thousands of participants and addressed the issue of whether or not omega-3 supplementation actually helps. That's a hot issue right now. Lots of doctors are promoting the idea that omega-3 deficiency has to be made up for with supplements. The study demonstrated that supplementation resulted in no benefits, found no reduced risk of total mortality or cardiovascular events in participants, and couldn't rule out an increased risk of cancer.[9] That's a powerful study that supports my premise: you can't make up for your dietary indiscretions with supplements.

Then we have The Cochrane Collaboration. I like studies done by Cochrane because, again, it's one of the more independent groups out there. They do meta-analyses of previously published studies. It's hard to find people and groups that aren't corrupted by industry influence in some form or another. This is a huge study: sixty-seven randomized trials, with close to a quarter of a million participants. And the researchers concluded as follows:

[N]o evidence to support antioxidant supplements for primary or secondary prevention. Vitamin A, beta-carotene, and vitamin

E may increase mortality. . . . Antioxidant supplements need to be considered medicinal products and should undergo sufficient evaluation before marketing.[10]

And people are just flabbergasted at this kind of stuff. You mean vitamin C and vitamin E might have medicinal properties, and I should be careful about taking them? Well, yes, a quarter of a million people in sixty-seven randomized, controlled trials is a pretty good sample. I don't think we can fault them for not having a large enough cohort here.

Then there's the Folate After Coronary Intervention Trial,[11] a study published in the *New England Journal of Medicine* in 2004. This study took patients who already had stents implanted and randomized them into two groups: one got folic acid; the other received a placebo. After six months, the results were clear: those getting the folic acid had their arteries clogging again faster than the others. The big take-home point here is that supplements should be treated like medicine. In that regard, they can be useful for specific and targeted purposes. But if you're self-medicating by buying this stuff over the Internet, through your neighbor in a multilevel marketing business, or at a health food store, and you're thinking that the worst-case scenario is ending up with expensive urine, you're wrong. People really need to rethink the money they spend on supplements and the potential damage to their health the supplements can cause.

GM: When you talk about expensive urine, I've often wondered how much of these supplements are just excreted?

PP: Well, a lot of it is excreted. But excreting substances not needed by the body can cause health issues, ranging from kidney stress to increasing risk of disease. The Folate After Intervention Trial showed that patients taking folic acid after angioplasty were developing arterial thickening faster than patients taking a placebo. The study was ended early as a result.

And there really is no such thing as a "natural" vitamin. In whole foods, nutrients are all bundled up in packages with coenzymes, conutrients, and that sort of thing. We purify these nutrients and take them in pill form, but the first thing the body starts doing is drawing cofactors out of the cell's tissues to try to create a complex that looks familiar. We've seen people develop what I call compensatory deficiencies. A person will take highly purified isolated nutrients and in the body's attempts to find something to do with these nutrients, it will actually deplete stores of other nutrients.

GM: So you're saying the body doesn't really know what to do with a dose of isolated vitamin E or isolated ascorbic acid?

PP: Right. The other problem you encounter is flooding the receptors. For example, there are about six hundred different carotenoids in foods. So you take in a massive dose of beta-carotene, for example, and that's one out of the six hundred. Well, you only have one carotenoid receptor in every cell, so you overwhelm the cells with this massive amount of beta-carotene you're taking in every day. Then you start eating actual food and your body can't use the other carotenoids you're taking in from the foods that you're eating.

GM: How about someone who takes the attitude, "Well, I'll pop a multivitamin once a day or once a week just in case I'm missing some nutrients somewhere that I don't know about." Still a bad idea?

PP: Well, the first thing I would do is laugh because nobody comes to The Wellness Forum with deficiency conditions. What, I wonder, do you think you're missing? And to my colleagues whom I meet at "alternative conferences," who tell me that they supplement their patients, I ask, "Why? When's the last time you had somebody in your office with scurvy? How many people in our line of work are treating beriberi these days?" All the people who are coming to us with health problems have diseases of excess. We're way too worried about deficiency in a place where deficiency is just not an issue. The second thing I ask people is, "Do you own stock in a vitamin company that you buy this stuff from?" I can't think of any other reason to take it. In other words, we don't have any evidence showing that this helps people in any way in the long term, so unless you own stock in the company and it's your way of supporting its efforts, I don't know why you'd want to waste your money.

GM: The one exception you make is with vitamin B_{12}, right?

PP: Yes, but it's very misunderstood because most people assume that as soon as you adopt a plant-based or vegan diet, B_{12} deficiency is an imminent risk. We see B_{12} deficiencies, and I do here, much more in meat eaters than we do in plant eaters. And the reason is, while they're taking in a lot of B_{12} in the animal foods that they're eating, they are notorious for having gastrointestinal problems, which range from simple constipation to serious inflammatory bowel diseases. A lot of times these people are deficient in intrinsic factor, which is a protein manufactured in the stomach that helps with the absorption and use of B_{12}. So you can be taking in plenty of B_{12} and not using it well at all. Having said that, most people who eat a plant-based or vegan diet are eating some fortified foods. We're consuming plant milks that are fortified with B_{12}, for example, and B_{12} requirements are really low. It's not very likely for somebody to develop a deficiency. The people most at risk are the rare individuals who eat no animal foods and no fortified foods. They *can* develop a B_{12} deficiency; supplements are probably a good idea for people like that.

191

Before I wrote my last book, I did some research looking for toxic effects of B_{12} and I couldn't find any. I don't discourage people who take a B_{12} supplement the way I discourage taking other supplements because you're not going to hurt yourself with it. So I'm fine with people saying that supplemental B_{12} is an insurance policy and they feel better for taking it.

GM: If the body doesn't know what to do with a massive dose of ascorbic acid or vitamin E, does it know how to process a sudden massive dose of B_{12}? Does the same problem present itself?

PP: Well, we don't really have any studies showing what happens when you take a massive dose of it.

GM: I don't mean a dose beyond what you would recommend, but five hundred micrograms is what my bottle says. It's five hundred micrograms of B_{12} that's been isolated, not integrated in food. Does the body know how to handle that?

PP: Yes, and here's kind of an interesting thing about B_{12} that's different from other supplements. B_{12} is bound to the protein in food and has to be separated from the protein by enzymes in the stomach; intrinsic factor helps a little bit with that. And when you take it in its supplement forms, it's already in what we call its free form, so it's actually pretty immediately useable. It's one situation where a supplement is actually easier to contend with than B_{12} in its natural form.

GM: What do clinical studies tell us about oils?

PP: They tell us that they're not health foods. This goes heavily against the grain of popular wisdom. There's a myth that it's not the amount of fat we're eating, but it's the type of fat; that olive oil is heart healthy and fish oil particularly heart healthy. Unfortunately, the evidence just doesn't take us there. In fact, oils can be successfully used to treat autoimmune conditions because they suppress immune function.[12] I don't think it's the right way to treat autoimmune conditions, but the fact they suppress immune function should tell a healthy person you don't want to be taking in a lot of this stuff.

I particularly like a study that Dr. David Blankenhorn did; he was looking at people consuming a "normal" diet versus those eating more of their fat as monounsaturated fat, which is what comes from olive oil, supposedly the healthy oil that we all want to include more of in our diet. It basically showed that the disease progressed just as much in those who consumed olive oil, high in the supposedly healthier monounsaturated fat, as it did in those who were consuming more saturated fat.[13] The study proves that people have got to ratchet the fat consumption down; they won't see any benefit by consuming olive oil instead of saturated fat in chicken or beef.

And we know that if people make dramatic, sweeping changes, they're more likely to stay compliant; that's been proven in clinical studies.

GM: Tell me about those studies.

PP: They're crucial studies. I can't tell you how many times over the years I've had people (many of them in health care) say to me, "Okay, let's assume you're right about how healthy this diet is. Nobody's going to do this. Even if you can get them to do it, they're not going to stick with it."

Dr. Neal Barnard did some early studies on Dr. Ornish's patients and found out their compliance levels were much higher than expected and they were much happier with their diets than the people eating the more moderate diet. He's also surveyed patients in his own studies to assess satisfaction and compliance on what we would think is a pretty strict diet and found the same thing. They're happier eating the stricter diet; they're happier with the results and they stay with it longer.

He did two of these studies, actually. One study showed that Dr. Ornish's patients were compliant on his diet to treat heart disease,[14] and another on diabetic patients.[15]

GM: More compliant than . . . ?

PP: More compliant than patients following dietary guidelines set by the American Heart Association or the American Diabetes Association. You see, if you're in the business of helping people change their diets, the specificity of the advice that you give becomes very important. Part of the problem with the diets recommended by our colleagues who stress moderation is that not only do they not work but their health status doesn't change. Our colleagues don't know what the heck they're talking about. Vague instructions about eating a little less of this or a little more of that are unclear and unworkable because "a little less" can mean something completely different to two different people. However, when people come here or they go to one of Barnard's programs or they're with Dr. Ornish or they're with Dr. McDougall, the directions are really specific. Now, you can choose to not follow them, but all of us are very clear in what we're saying to people, so they have a much easier time with implementation.

I can tell you from personal experience that people will stick with dietary instructions if they're presented with the right evidence, which is partly a matter of understanding the futility of what they're currently doing. We can get them to make the change, but, contrary to the conventional wisdom, if we get them to make the big sweeping change, they're much more likely to stick with the diet they've adopted. The reason is that big changes in diet bring about big changes in health; the changes are highly motivating. There's a clear discernible difference in their health and in their weight. Doctors are telling me all the time, "I tell people to alter their diet this way or that way; they try, but they don't stick with it." Well, that's because it seems like a whole lot of effort for not much return. But if you take a type 2 diabetic and put him on a diet that reverses his diabetes in two weeks, or if you take somebody with erectile dysfunction and you solve the problem in a matter of a month, those people aren't going to be as interested in cheeseburgers anymore. They see the results of the dietary changes they've made and it motivates them to stay compliant. And diet always brings results quicker than drugs.

GM: As studies prove?

PP: Absolutely. Diet changes work incredibly fast, as was initially demonstrated in a study done by Dr. James Anderson at the University of Kentucky. He did studies on diabetic patients using a low-fat, high-fiber, plant-based diet in the 1980s. He showed that in three weeks, type 1 diabetics could reduce insulin by 40 percent, cholesterol dropped by 30 percent, and twenty-four out of twenty-five type 2 diabetics were able to completely discontinue their insulin medication.[16] If you talk to endocrinologists who are using metformin or insulin or whatever combination of drugs they're using to treat diabetics, they can't get the treatment right in a three-week time period, let alone reverse the type 2 diabetes or reduce insulin needs in a type 1 inside three weeks. These are nothing short of miraculous results that cannot be duplicated with drugs. We've seen people have their cholesterol drop by eighty points in five days. You can't do that with a statin drug. And so not only is this diet better than the drugs from a health perspective but it's more effective than the drugs and works faster.

195

GM: Well, what do we know from studies about the effectiveness of drugs and surgical interventions for cardiovascular disease?

PP: There were three major studies that showed that surgical intervention was no better than drug therapy: the 1984 Veterans Administration Coronary Artery Bypass Surgery Cooperative Study Group;[17] the European Coronary Surgery Study Group of 1988;[18] and the Coronary Artery Surgery Study of 1990.[19] All three studies showed that the outcomes for patients who have bypass surgery versus patients who only take drugs are the same, with the exception of an advantage to the surgery group for those with damage to the left ventricle. There was also the AVERT study that showed that patients who did not receive angioplasty but took Lipitor experienced fewer heart attacks, less chest pain, and made fewer visits to the hospital.[20]

Angioplasty involves risk: often the inflating of the balloon releases plaque and causes heart attacks. And very often the arteries are blocked again within a few months of the procedure. Yet we spend billions of dollars a year on angioplasty.

The research shows that bypass surgery is really only warranted about 3 percent of the time—in those cases when doctors can get to somebody during or right after a myocardial infarction, or when there's extensive damage to the left ventricle. Other than that, it's a totally voluntary and useless surgery that costs about $100,000 over a five-year period for the surgery and follow-up care.

When we consider how useless these surgical interventions generally are, we need to factor in that about twenty thousand people per year die as a result of angioplasty[21] and another ten thousand die as a result of bypass surgery.[22] It's unconscionable that this practice continues. So the question comes up, and I've asked it of Dr. Esselstyn, "Why do we keep doing this?" He says, "Well, Pam, somebody's got to pay for these cardiac cathedrals that they build." The average hospital, after all, thrives on bypass and angioplasty. So it's the unwitting patients and their insurance companies who wind up paying.

GM: We've talked about studies that show that surgical intervention for cardiovascular disease is generally no more effective than drug therapy. But exactly how effective is drug therapy?

PP: Not much at all. We have many studies that show that cholesterol-lowering drugs don't significantly reduce the risk of heart attack, stroke, or death. So why would someone take a useless drug unless he has stock in Merck and feels like he ought to support the cause? No one should want to take these drugs. In fact, the package inserts on the drugs pretty much say that in small print; Crestor is one. The prescribing information states that Crestor reduces the risk of major cardiovascular events by 1.2 percent.[23] That's not much of a risk reduction, particularly when factoring in the side effects. So it will lower cholesterol levels, but it's not very effective for actually solving the problem. What it will do is help a person die with good blood work.

GM: It seems to me such a powerful, provocative statement to say that cholesterol-lowering medication doesn't reduce the risk of death. How does that affect a nation of doctors who are prescribing such drugs? Do they realize it's not reducing the risk of death or serious events? Do they accept that?

PP: A lot of them do. But so many doctors get their information from drug reps and through continuing medical education programs sponsored by drug companies. This, combined with the fact that many don't read medical journals regularly and don't know how to interpret the results of the articles they do read, is why so many patients get bad advice from doctors.

GM: When my mother was about seventy years old, my parents moved to Florida. She had suffered from angina since her mid-fifties and after seeing her, my mother's new cardiologist immediately recommended she have an angioplasty. Luckily, my father, who was always skeptical of the medical profession, was in the office with her and said, "Well, you could do that, honey; it's your heart, after all. Just keep in mind that if you do it, I'm going to leave you." So there was a big fight in the doctor's office with the doctor saying, "Who are you going to listen to, him or me? What does he know about medicine? If you're going to listen to him, then you're fired. I don't want you as a patient!" Well, my parents had been happily married for more than forty years. My mother obviously didn't want to get divorced, so she refused the intervention, the doctor fired my mother, and she never went back to him. She's ninety-three years old today and has never had a heart attack or any cardiac event. I've got her on a low-fat, plant-based diet; she'll probably outlive that cardiologist.

PP: I always find it interesting when doctors fire patients. It's despicable. Basically, what the doctor is saying is, "You'll do as you're told. I'm not interested in having you as a patient if you decide to have an original thought or become proactive on your own behalf." They don't say it in those words, but that's the essence of what they're communicating.

IT'S THE FOOD, STUPID

. . . .

GM: Pam, we've talked a lot about individual dietary choices and their effect on human health. But there are also collective choices we make as a society that influence health in all kinds of ways, not least by directing, or misdirecting, the citizenry in making their individual choices. So let's discuss public policy and propose some changes to the status quo.

PP: Well, public policy has to change because we simply cannot afford to keep spending as much as we spend on health care and expect to have either a vibrant economy or a balanced budget. It's simply impossible. We spent $8,000 per person on health care services in 2009, the most of any country in the world by a long shot. Poor Norway limped along in second place at $5,000 per person. So we're spending 60 percent more than the second most expensive health care system in the world.[1] That's insane, particularly for a country that ranks thirty-sixth in the world in longevity. If a company made laptops and it was spending 60 percent more for microprocessors and other parts than its competitors, and yet its laptops came in thirty-sixth in a test for durability, I don't think that company would be in business very long.

GM: When I think of our health care system, I'm reminded of what my doctor said to me once. As I mentioned, he's got a humble approach to his practice, which is why I return to him annually. He said, "I'm not interested in the practice of health care. I'm interested in the practice of medicine." I asked him what the difference was. He told me that he sees health care as the system that doctors get caught up in: he has to see so many patients per hour, deal with the insurance companies, diagnose and treat according to guidelines, etc. He's dismissive, to put it mildly, of the health care system. He's passionate about the practice of medicine; medicine to him means a lot of talking and listening, getting to know his patients, and treating them as individual human beings. He happens to believe in colonoscopy screening, but when I turn it down annually, he hears me out and he's fine with that.

PP: The problem is medical education. There are plenty of doctors who have the best of intentions, but they've never been schooled in nutrition. If they're seeing patients with degenerative diseases and they're not practicing nutrition, they're not practicing medicine, period.

Doctors are taught to mitigate and treat symptoms. We need to set the bar higher in training health care professionals. Health care has to become outcome-oriented. We have to teach doctors that stopping the progression of diseases, and even reversing diseases, is an option.

GM: How do we do that?

PP: Be the first one to show up in your doctor's office reversing disease with diet. Doctors were never taught in school that you can eat your way out of disease. However, be your doctor's first patient who does, and maybe your doctor will take a fresh look at diet as an intervention tool. Until medical schools give doctors a proper education, patients may have to do it.

GM: And then there's the education of the rest of us. The schools are key to getting children off to a healthy start in life, yet school nutrition guidelines are effectively written by agribusinesses through their shills in the U.S. Department of Agriculture (USDA). What can be done to help kids eat healthy lunches in schools?

PP: Well, first, of course, if you can pack a healthy lunch for your child that's generally best, but that's not an option for everyone. We need to concern ourselves with what's offered in the cafeteria. The federal nutrition guidelines allow for meals that are 30 percent fat, which is a good way to promote obesity, and it's been quite effective at doing just that.

GM: In fact, the problem is even worse than those obscene guidelines, because in 2005 only 30 percent of schools met the guidelines for maximum saturated fat allowed in school lunches.[2] So first they set preposterously unhealthy guidelines and then find even those lax guidelines too onerous to meet, so they violate them with impunity. They're making children obese and diabetic and sick in countless ways, and we know that obese children and adolescents often become obese adults. So the degree of failure here, both moral and nutritional, is stunning.

Representative Jared Polis of Colorado, a rare congressman who's aware of these issues, introduced The Healthy School Meals

Act of 2010, for which the Physicians Committee for Responsible Medicine (PCRM) is fighting the good fight. This would be only a first step, but a terrific first step, toward improving school nutrition. It would increase the availability of plant-based foods in schools, incentivize schools to provide plant-based options, such as plant milks, and remove the restrictions currently in place for non-dairy milks. Children would no longer have to bring in a note from their doctor explaining why they don't choose to drink bovine lactation fluid. Unfortunately, the bill may not have a chance to be voted on until the Child Nutrition Act next comes up for renewal in 2015. But in the meantime, before the government acts, parents and even children have to take matters into their own hands.

PP: Right. One of the reasons why our own foundation's focus is at the local level is that a great deal of authority has been taken away from the local school or school system, but not so much that a group of concerned parents, teachers, or students can't make substantive changes in their local schools. If you want better lunches for your kid, you can start gathering a group of interested people who can begin to put pressure on the school system to set up a committee to get this done. You don't want to focus on getting all the unhealthy foods, like cow's milk, out of the school because that's not likely to happen any time soon; instead, you want to focus on insisting that healthy alternatives be made available. A salad bar, at least one low-fat vegan option, and a plant milk should be offered every day. This would make life easier for the nutritionally aware parent who now won't be forced to prepare a lunch every day, and it would expose all the children, whether their parents have a consciousness around these issues or not, to some healthy choices. People shouldn't feel hopeless and powerless at the local level; that's where the most immediate solutions are available.

GM: Let's say there's a high school kid who's on the diet we recommend, and he would like to have new kinds of food choices in the cafeteria. What should he do?

PP: Let me tell you the story of a very exclusive private school here in Columbus. A group of students got together and sent a letter to the headmaster. They wrote something like this: "We get a great education here. We have unparalleled opportunities and we appreciate that. Our facilities are second to none." And they went on with praise. And then they said, "But there's one area in which we feel that the school has not paid much attention to—it's not up to par with the rest of what goes on here—and that is the food that's served in the cafeteria. We think that an educational institution that strives for excellence everywhere should pay as much attention to this issue as to academics." It was a very well-crafted, polite letter; I was astounded that it came from high school students. After it stimulated some parents to get active on the issue, changes were made in the cafeteria. Now, that was in a private school. You can imagine that with tuition bills being as high as they are, private school administrators are likely to show responsiveness to the concerns of parents and students.

I have another example from a public school situation. I met a young woman whose mother had converted to a plant-based diet for health reasons. She got into it after her mom and discovered that there was nothing for her to eat at school. She started asking why. She spoke to the people who were running the cafeteria and was told, essentially, "That's just the way things are." She refused to accept that, so, as a sophomore in high school, she started a campaign that actually resulted in changes in the cafeteria. I think that kids can make a big difference because when kids initiate a campaign for healthy food, that immediately overcomes the argument that the advocates for the status quo constantly bring up, which is that kids won't eat healthy food. Well, present a letter

signed by two hundred kids saying, "We want healthy food," and they can't use that easy, thoughtless excuse anymore.

Let's keep in mind, too, that high school is supposed to be about getting kids to think critically. So why not get them to think critically about something that's critically important, like their health? We ought to be assigning kids comparative research on health issues. For example, give them the assignment to research the question, "Is cow's milk good for you or bad for you?" Give them a dozen websites to visit, equally divided between those that do and do not advocate consumption of cow's milk, and let the kids prepare their findings and offer their own opinions. They can weigh the opinions expressed by PCRM against those offered by the American Diabetes Association. I don't think you'd find too much pushback on that idea. I don't think a lot of parents are going to protest, "Forcing my kid to do research is a bad idea." We can be considerably more adventurous in a high school classroom than in a grade school classroom, and we should be.

GM: So we should invite kids to actually think about their health?

PP: Absolutely. That's going to pay dividends in untold ways. I have every confidence that high school students who research these issues will wind up, more often than not, making better choices for their health. I bet they will also wind up knowing more about nutrition than their doctors.

GM: Hospitals, like schools, are sometimes public and sometimes private institutions, but it seems to be the case that hospital food is almost universally atrocious.

PP: Hospitals are run by health care professionals; we have to train health care professionals about diet. If you or I walked down the halls of a hospital, we'd be appalled at the food served:

meatloaf, eggs and bacon, greasy pancakes and butter, chicken and turkey, and macaroni and cheese served to people who've had heart attacks and strokes. Now, if someone came to the hospital for emphysema, they wouldn't be offered cigarettes. However, if they come in for any number of medical conditions, they're served the very foods that caused them. Yet doctor after doctor, nurse after nurse, and dietitian after dietitian walk down the halls of a hospital and see patients eating these meals that are counter-productive to their recovery. By doing nothing about it, they are essentially saying, "This is okay with me!"

GM: What would happen if doctors, nurses, and dietitians told hospital administrators, "We can't feed people like this."

PP: If enough of them spoke up, I believe that it would change overnight. In the meantime, patients need to complain and bring in healthy food from the outside. And if you're bringing in food from the outside, I suggest you negotiate with the hospital to reduce the bill, since there's no reason you should pay for food that, for your own good, you refuse to eat.

GM: I read an article recently about film director Duncan Roy, who was wrongly imprisoned in the Los Angeles Men's Central Jail for a period of months, in which he said, "People in that jail are hungry, and nobody gives a damn."[3] I don't think prison food is something the general population cares a lot about, but it's not hard to imagine that the facts, if reported, would be Dickensian. What could or should be done about prison food?

PP: Dr. Antonia Demas is a friend of mine who did a remarkably low-cost project in Miami at the Bay Point School, a residential school for violent male juvenile offenders. She recruited a group of kids and asked them to eat a plant-based diet, to participate in the preparation of the food, and to keep a journal while they were engaged in the project. And the kids started getting better grades, their health improved, their athleticism improved, and their behavior improved.[4] She brought to one of our conferences excerpts from their journals with their names redacted. In the beginning of one of the journals, the writing was so bad you could hardly read or understand it. And then, thirty-five pages in, the kid's writing is completely legible, the grammar has changed, the sentences are finished, the thoughts are clear, and the statements were amazing.

GM: Is the implication that the diet itself is improving clarity of mind?

PP: Oh, absolutely. This is explainable from a medical perspective because we know that the brain is a huge user of water, oxygen, and glucose. When you don't eat well, it's not just that you're not fueling your body—you're not fueling your brain. When people eat the food that their bodies are designed to eat, they think more clearly, they are able to participate in life better, and they make better decisions. I remember one kid wrote in his journal about how one of the benefits of this experience was that he would one day be able to make healthy food for his wife and his family. Now, for a juvenile offender to have positive thoughts like that toward women and family because he's been exposed, in a caring way, to a diet that helps people care for themselves, speaks volumes.

I think a lot of people would perceive feeding prisoners a good diet as providing them with an undeserved luxury. Actually, I think the people who would benefit most would be society at large. The guards and the wardens would certainly have an easier time and we would return prisoners back to society as more productive people.

GM: I don't see why even those who have a "tough love" attitude toward prisoners would object to feeding them very plain, simple, inexpensive foods like oatmeal, rice and beans, potatoes, corn, wheat, fruits, and vegetables. Prisoners certainly shouldn't go hungry, so let's feed them inexpensive, filling, starchy foods. None of the rich foods of royalty, like meat and fish and cheese. Why the hell would we feed meat and dairy, which require so much energy, water, and cost to produce, to people who have presumably committed crimes? Let's put them on an inexpensive, low-fat, starch-based, plant-based diet; they'll wind up being the healthiest population in the country. Shouldn't this idea appeal to both conservatives and liberals? Let's "punish" prisoners with cheap food that makes them healthy. And since they're wards of the state, when they get healthy, that saves the taxpayers money.

PP: Meat and dairy, unfortunately, aren't as expensive as they should be. That's the result of another public policy—farm subsidies.

GM: And you'd favor ending them outright?

PP: Yeah, let's get rid of them.

GM: I'd be fine with either of two outcomes. The first is the cleanest: get rid of all farm subsidies, as you say. Get government out of the business of picking the winners in agriculture—and it has effectively picked large-scale, animal agriculture interests—and turn it into a free market. Again, that's an idea that should appeal to conservatives. I'd also be fine with subsidizing only crops raised organically and intended for human beings, not animals. Then at least our tax dollars would be helping farmers help the population get healthier, while incentivizing stewardship of the land.

207

PP: The reason why it's best to get government out of this completely, and you and I may have some philosophical differences on this score, is that I don't think that government generally solves problems; I think more often it creates them. Once you propose that we're going to subsidize this instead of that, who's going to decide what to subsidize? How is that decision going to get made in a way that isn't effectively corrupt? We cannot afford to continue to grow government. We cannot afford to continue to keep throwing money at problems. We can't just build another USDA down the street staffed with different people who subsidize different farm crops and magically find a way to pay for it. We're done. I'm all for government simply getting out of that business.

GM: That would be more than fine with me. Another activity that perhaps the government should consider exiting is the business of issuing nutritional guidelines.

PP: Absolutely. USDA has screwed it up beyond recognition and it's not a productive use of the agency's time. We've already discussed the problems with industry and agriculture influencing the USDA, but in preparation for a class that I teach, I visited the websites of a number of other countries that issue dietary guidelines. I spoke in South Africa last year, so I went to the South African government's website where it promotes dietary guidelines. I've looked at Australia and several different countries.

GM: Is any country doing a good job of it?

PP: No, and for very familiar reasons—they're pressured by the same political influences from food and agricultural groups that we are here. If we can't find a model government policy anywhere on the planet that manages to eliminate this level of influence and provide impartial information to the public, maybe we should just get the government out of the dietary recommendations business. It can't be any worse than the status quo.

GM: Actually, I hope you're right about that last point, but I wonder: As misguided as the current guidelines are, if there were no guidelines at all for school lunchrooms, would some states begin serving children meals that are 50 to 60 percent fat? In other words, are we better off with lousy guidelines that are the product of tacit corruption, or no guidelines at all? It's a head-scratcher for me.

I think I'd favor retaining a role for government in issuing guidelines, but moving it from the USDA to the surgeon general's office. And then all we'd have to do would be to get Dr. John McDougall or Dr. Neal Barnard appointed surgeon general and we're good.

PP: If we could be guaranteed that these men or someone like them would be in that position, I'd be all for it. The problem is there are only a few doctors in the country who understand these issues and are capable, in my opinion, of doing the right thing. The likelihood that one of them would be appointed is not great. In fact, a few years ago, PCRM resolved to influence the appointment to the Dietary Guidelines Advisory Committee of some nutrition professionals with no ties to industry. PCRM submitted several highly qualified names; not one was appointed. Given its track record, we're better off getting government out of it.

GM: The other guidelines that are crucial to consumers are the labeling laws that govern what is written on the packages of food we buy. Bold health claims are made about various types of foods, and the nutrition labels can be confusing. What should be done?

PP: The most important thing that we could do would meet opposition from food manufacturers, but it would be a simple law to draft and pass. The law would simply tell manufacturers of foods that the only thing they can do is put the ingredients on the label. In other words, a manufacturer can say it's delicious and it smells great, but it can't make any nutritional or health claims about the product. That would stop all this silly game-playing in which manufacturers take a stick of margarine that's 100 percent fat, fortify it with plant sterols, and say it's good for lowering cholesterol. The next thing I'd recommend doing would be to reduce the nutrition facts label to the basics: calories and calories from fat. That's it.

GM: What about people who need to restrict sodium? Shouldn't they know how much sodium is in a given food? Or, for the sugar-sensitive, how many grams of sugar are in food? Or cholesterol content?

PP: Sodium would be listed in the ingredients list, as would animal foods. We teach our members to pay attention only to the ingredients list and to avoid products with long lists of ingredients, many of which are not recognizable as food. It works.

GM: Medicare remains the most debated, the most complex, and certainly the most fiscally significant public health policy issue. It's easy to imagine someone writing a scholarly tome exploring all the complexities of the program and analyzing in a thousand pages a raft of competing ideas on how to keep it afloat. Not so easy to imagine anyone actually reading that book. Meanwhile, journalists and policy wonks debate the issue endlessly, politicians rant and rave and posture, and nothing gets done. So, to save everyone a mountain of time and trouble, and to save the country from tens of trillions in increased deficit spending in the coming

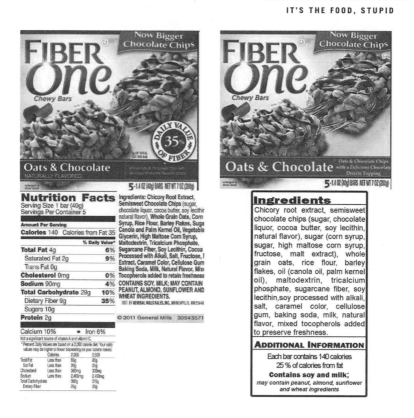

Labels should be simple and easy to read. The current, complicated label system costs a fortune as federal agencies are forced to spend time reviewing labels, policing manufacturers, and responding to lawsuits filed by manufacturers over claims that are denied. And consumers are still left with a label that few people pay attention to and many don't know how to interpret.

On the left is the front and back of the package of a popular product. On the right is my proposed version. Since no health claims would be allowed if my rules were adopted, the front of the box would not mislead people into thinking that this product promotes good health because of its fiber content (the fiber is due to added fiber from chicory root, not because the ingredients are high in fiber), and the term "naturally flavored" would not be permitted.

"Nutrition Facts" charts would not appear on the back of the box, which would prevent misrepresentation about the amount of fiber. Sugars and oils would be grouped together, making it easier for consumers to see just how much of these ingredients are in the product.

With this simpler label, consumers would readily see that the front of the box shows essentially a picture of a candy bar, and the ingredients list is consistent with a candy bar. Some consumers would still buy it because it tastes good, but more would not consider it a health food.

211

decades, I say that we try to solve the problem in a few minutes here.

PP: Happy to help.

GM: Medicare's fiscal nightmare looms because of a combination of factors:

1. Demographics, with an aging generation of baby boomers (eighty million people will be on Medicare by 2040);
2. A sick and obese population of seniors made unhealthy by unhealthy food; and
3. A health care system geared toward incessant, expensive testing, often followed by expensive intervention.

As we know, high-tech medical intervention doesn't always lead to better health outcomes, but it does always lead to higher costs; in the case of Medicare, those costs are borne by the taxpayers. The trend is unsustainable, to say the least.

I believe a decent society provides its senior citizens with an affordable, accessible system of medical care. I don't want Americans to lose the Medicare entitlement. But it's simply unsustainable on the present path. So here's my suggestion: society should have a pact with its senior citizens. If you've paid into Medicare during your working life, we will take care of you in your retirement years. If you're sick, Medicare will continue to cover your costs if you need to go to the doctor or the hospital. But an endless hunt for medical problems should not be part of that compact. Nor should most interventions consequent to that hunt. If you're a senior citizen and you for some reason want a "preventive" colonoscopy or mammogram or stress test or angiogram or prostate-specific antigen test or vitamin D test or EKG or Dexa scan, it should be on your dime. If you are asymptomatic, but your preventive testing leads to an intervention (other than removal of a tumor or polyp), let that be on your dime, too. If we end Medicare as a discretionary testing benefit, we may save enough money to keep the program solvent for many more years. And I suspect it'll save lives as well.

My parents had a very good friend who was about ninety years old. She went to a doctor complaining of chest pain, so the doctor proposed an angiogram. During the procedure, they nicked her aorta and she died a few days later. It's unconscionable. They could have just put her on a low-fat, plant-based diet, but instead they killed her, and charged it to the taxpayers.

When my father, who at this point was a frail old man in his late eighties with Parkinson's disease dementia, passed out at home, we made the mistake of calling 911. The medics took him to the hospital, where he remained for a week, ostensibly to combat his orthostatic hypotension. They ran every test on him imaginable. He was a frail, dying old man who didn't even know what state he was in—when asked that question by his neurologist, I swear he said "confusion"—but the one thing he knew was that he wanted to get out of the hospital. They ran one test after another on him and billed the taxpayers $70,000 for it. They still didn't stabilize his blood pressure, but they did give him a urinary tract infection from the catheter. I was wracked with guilt for putting him in the hospital. So the next time he passed out, we kept him home and took care of him until he came to. One thing I'm proud of is that we allowed him to die at home; he never saw a hospital again.

PP: The disturbing fact is that the overtesting and overtreating we've discussed before is especially targeted at the senior population. The situations you described with your family and family friend are not isolated incidents.

Neil Armstrong died as a result of complications of bypass surgery at the age of eighty-two. As I mentioned before, only a tiny fraction of bypass surgeries in the United States are medically warranted; the procedure is even less useful and more dangerous in people over the age of eighty.[5] But after a routine stress test that Armstrong failed, he underwent a quadruple bypass. Although we'll most likely never know the details of the conversation he had with his cardiologist, I would be willing to bet that the discussion did not include the recommendation to adopt a low-fat, plant-based diet or a recommendation to read Dr. Caldwell Esselstyn's book, both far less expensive alternatives to bypass surgery. It would be hard to believe that Armstrong would have opted for bypass had he been informed properly of the risks and minimal benefits of the procedure and the potential benefits of plant-based nutrition.

GM: Pam, how would you save Medicare?

PP: The way to make Medicare sustainable is to stop paying for tests and procedures that have no basis in science. You mentioned before that society should take care of health care for its seniors. I agree. Here's how we could do it in a way that would have a positive effect on all payers. We should incorporate the findings of independent research groups like Cochrane into the decision-making process. For example, Cochrane's research, which is extensive, shows that mammograms are inadvisable for any group. For every woman saved, six women die unnecessarily. Neither Medicare nor any other entity should pay for mammograms. If you want a mammogram, you can pay for it yourself, but neither the government nor insurance companies should pay for those tests. Same with Dexa scans, PSA testing, colonoscopy, and other diagnostic tests. And the same would hold true for treatments. If Avastin does not add a single day of survival for breast cancer patients, it simply would not be reimbursable. You could pay for it yourself if you were convinced you wanted it.

Independent groups like Cochrane should be hired to conduct research on tests, drugs, and procedures to determine which are worthwhile. Congress and any bureaucracy susceptible to political influence should be kept out of the discussion. The National Institutes of Health at one point convened a panel that concluded that breast cancer screening should not be a blanket recommendation based on the evidence; Congress overrode the scientists and overturned the panel's recommendations.[6] This should be unacceptable.

If we develop a system that relies on evidence, instead of confining our discussion only to who should pay for any test or intervention that any doctor orders or any patient wants, we could contain costs, which would free up enough money to provide scientifically justified care to all seniors. Doctors and hospitals have a financial incentive to preserve the status quo, but we know that the status quo is terrible health outcomes at unsustainable cost.

GM: Are you optimistic that government will reform itself and make these kinds of changes happen?

PP: No, but I think we can educate the public one person at a time, until so many people have dropped out of the system that the system does not exist in its current form. The only workable solution to our Medicare problem and our larger health care cost problem is to reduce demand for health services. The ways to do that are to create a healthier and better-informed populace and to demand that science, not a profit-oriented medical establishment, determines what is worth paying for.

GM: Since we did such a good job of developing a plan for Medicare, let's help balance the budget. We raise and kill more than ten billion land animals a year in America, and kill another fifty-three billion aquatic animals.[7] If we were to tax this carnage at an average of only about a dollar per animal—considerably more for the large mammals and considerably less for the sardines—with the tax burden shared by the producers and the slaughterhouses and the commercial fisheries, that would generate about $60 billion per year for the Treasury. Some of that money could then be dedicated to remediating the environmental damage to the land and rivers brought on by animal agriculture. Of course, the argument would be made that such a tax on producers would be passed along to the consumer. To the extent that that's true, it would only increase prices on foods that are making Americans sick, thereby discouraging their consumption, and leading to reduced medical costs, a further savings to the government, and a boost to the economy generally. So, while I don't believe it's on anyone's radar, theoretically a slaughterhouse and fisheries tax would be a superb way to raise revenues for a government awash in red ink.

PP: I agree. Those who pollute the water supply and destroy the environment should be responsible for paying for it. And the price of animal products should have some bearing on the true cost of producing them, which includes this damage.

GM: New York City Mayor Michael Bloomberg has been in the news in the last few years, first banning trans fats from restaurants, then banning sodas and sugary drinks larger than sixteen ounces from restaurants, movie theaters, and street carts. Some are attacking the mayor for acting like Big Brother. What's your opinion of his initiatives?

PP: We live in America, not China. I worry about who is going to make up the food police and what guidelines they are going to use. If we're going to let Mayor Bloomberg decide the size of the soft drinks and whether or not trans fat is allowed . . . well, what if Mayor Bloomberg talks to Dr. Barry Sears, who tells him that baked potatoes are bad for you? Is that the next food we're going to eliminate? The more government gets involved, the more messed up things get.

GM: I grant your logic, but all the same, I support the mayor's actions. It might not be the most sensible or ideologically consistent way to improve public health, but when you're in a crisis of the proportions that we face, I appreciate that at least somebody in a position of power is trying to do *something*. More than a dozen other state and local governments have emulated Mayor Bloomberg's ban on trans fats, and it appears to have changed eating habits in NYC, at least slightly for the better.[8] And while it seems silly to ban sugary drinks larger than sixteen ounces while allowing consumers to buy three eight-ounce sugary drinks, I'll welcome it for the attention it brings to the issue.

PP: I'll continue to disagree. Growing the problem, as in more regulation, does not make it better. As Albert Einstein once said, "You cannot solve a problem with the same thinking that created it." A major contributor to our health care crisis is government; let's get it out of the picture, instead of rearranging it.

GM: Personally, I wouldn't object if Mayor Bloomberg were to really show some guts and tax cheeseburgers. They clearly cause even more damage to people's health than giant soft drinks. In fact, I have a theory that Obama's presidency was nearly destroyed by the cheeseburger.

PP: I'm also very anti-cheeseburger, but could you explain that one?

GM: Sure. When Obama first ran for president, I agreed with him on most of the issues, but I had one quibble: he kept eating cheeseburgers at his photo ops. Proof that he was a regular Joe, even if his name was Barack. Well, I certainly wasn't going to let his dietary indiscretions keep me from supporting him, so I thought of it as a quibble without consequence. But it was indicative of his lack of understanding of health, and his tendency to conflate health with health insurance.

Imagine an Iraqi bureaucrat at the worst point in the insurgency in 2004, with car bombs exploding in markets all over Baghdad, and IEDs blowing up American Humvees. The bureaucrat surveys the carnage around him and has a "Eureka!" moment: "What this city needs is car insurance reform."

That's precisely how Obama has approached the atrocity that is the state of American health. Our real problem isn't the large number of uninsured, lamentable as that fact may be. Our real problems are obesity, diabetes, heart disease, cancer, and all the other ailments that come from eating foods like the cheeseburger that our president is so delighted to chomp down on at photo ops. Obesity is so widespread that he apparently couldn't find anyone to be surgeon general who wasn't obese. So I realize now that what those cheeseburger photo ops really demonstrated is that the man knows nothing about health. And knowing nothing about health allowed him to believe that having health insurance is a matter of greater significance than having the real thing, health. The Affordable Care Act, his signature achievement, has nothing whatsoever to do with health.

PP: I want to say first of all that it's not entirely his fault. There is a tendency for the market to pay attention to who's paying for health care versus whether there might be a way to obviate the need for those services in the first place. He's caught up in a system that emphasizes who's going to pay, instead of whether there's another way to provide care, so it's not entirely his fault.

What is his fault is that, in spite of public sentiment against it, the bill passed anyway. It's very difficult to manage any situation that involves significant change with zero buy-in from the public.

GM: As a Democrat, I agree with you.

PP: I don't find many who don't. This is not a partisan issue; this isn't Republicans against Democrats; this is practicality setting in. It doesn't matter if you're Republican or Democrat; if you have a simple grasp of economics, you'll understand that if a breast cancer patient diagnosed yesterday pays her first $175 health premium today and then sucks up $50,000 worth of care, you can't have a whole lot of that going on before it becomes unsustainable. We can't print money at the insurance companies. So this is a bad piece of legislation that will eventually have to be dismantled, at least in part.

In government, we have to be very careful of the law of unintended consequences. We need to think through all the things that will happen as a by-product of a new law, outcomes that were never intended. The more people, and especially businesspeople, understand the Affordable Care Act, the more they will object to it. When that happens, the federal government will have to make more exceptions to keep disaster from happening. And that's where all these exceptions come in—

GM: Yeah, all these waivers to businesses to sidestep the law.

PP: Oh, they will have to keep doing it. I read a survey recently where this polling company called CEOs to say, "We're not going to use your name, but if this law stands, will you drop your health insurance?" And some alarming percentage of CEOs said, "We wouldn't be the first but we would be a fast second." In other words, all we need is one large company to drop coverage and the dominoes will start to fall. I think that the government cannot afford to have a major player say, "We give up. We're not going to provide insurance at our company anymore." So they've granted all these waivers trying to keep the ship from sinking and they can't keep doing that but then again they have no choice.

GM: It's like getting special dispensations from the pope. It's an absurd way to create national policy. And let's not forget that while Chief Justice John Roberts upheld the mandate's constitutionality as a tax, he also struck down the law's enforcement provisions to effectively compel the states to expand the Medicaid program, the mechanism by which roughly 15 million more people were to obtain health insurance. So the law will not bring us anywhere near universal coverage, in spite of the mandate. I do approve of the law's provisions for government-sponsored insurance (the preexisting condition insurance plan) for those who are refused coverage by private insurers, but that was a nice, simple provision that didn't require a mandate. Unfortunately, it's going to be replaced by the more complex exchanges in 2014.

The absurd mandate has been posited by almost every commentator in the media, with the notable exception of Lawrence O'Donnell, as the *sine qua non* of Obamacare. The truth is that it's a sham and a mirage, a toothless response to the largely imaginary problem of people "gaming the system" by going to the emergency room for a cold. In fact, people don't fail to buy health insurance because they want to "game the system"; they fail to buy it either because they can't afford it or because they feel they don't need it. There is no enforcement mechanism for the mandate. What happens if you don't buy health insurance as mandated by the law? You get fined—$95 the first year, or 1 percent of your income. What happens if you don't pay the fine? Nothing. There's no penalty for not paying the fine. Here's what the law says: "In the case of any failure by a taxpayer to timely pay any penalty imposed by this section, such taxpayer shall not be subject to any criminal prosecution or penalty with respect to such payer." So if the mandate is a violation of constitutional freedoms, as some passionately argue, it's only a symbolic one; in a very real, practical sense, it's merely an invitation to break the law. That doesn't strike me as wise policy.

PP: No, it's not, but I'll tell you what I think the take-home message is for anyone who is reading this book, regardless of her political convictions. Whether you are sick or healthy, whether you have health insurance or not, whether you are a Republican or a Democrat, the bottom line is the same. You have to take responsibility for your own health. You've got to get the information that you need to make informed choices about health care. It doesn't really matter who's going to pay for it; it doesn't really matter whether Obamacare stands or doesn't stand. If it got erased tomorrow, and we went back to the way it was two years ago, the person with coronary artery disease faces the same choice: he can either do what his doctors tell him, which is not medically warranted or scientifically supported, or he can take matters into his own hands and find his own solution. If you are perfectly healthy and you want to stay that way, you're not going to stay that way listening to most of the authorities who you generally might seek out for advice about such things. You've got to drop out of the system and look for alternative options. And when I say alternative, I don't mean "alternative medicine"; I mean alternatives to all traditional health care.

You can go visit doctors, do what you're told, and keep eating what's advertised on television and what's served in fast-food joints and restaurants. Or you can drop out of all of that and take care of yourself. If enough people do that, we won't have to worry about who's paying for health care anymore because we're going to get rid of so much of this health care cost that it'll be a nonissue.

GM: I confronted Michael Moore on this recently at a public event in Los Angeles. Again, I'm a left-wing guy and I've admired several of his films, but not *Sicko*, because, as I told him, he doesn't understand anything about health. His overriding issue is that fifty million Americans don't have insurance coverage and he made the point that fifty thousand people died last year because they couldn't afford medical care. Now if that's true, it's of course indefensible.

PP: It is, but more people died from too much medical intervention.

GM: I pointed that out to him. Probably at least five times as many people died because they had excessive and unnecessary and bad medical care. He didn't have a response to that. He was sitting on the stage, all three hundred or so pounds of him, arguing that we should have Medicare for all. So in other words, people should be free to eat hot dogs and pizza and cheeseburgers and then force us to do unlimited medical testing on them and provide unlimited surgical interventions, with the government picking up the tab. *That's* the progressive solution? What exactly is progressive about bankrupting the country so that Michael Moore can have as many angioplasties as his cardiologist recommends? What's progressive about bankrupting government so that it won't have any money to spend on education, clean energy, infrastructure, the environment, and all of the other things that Michael Moore and I believe in?

PP: Health care costs are going to strangle our economy if we don't put a limit on them. What the government seems to want to do is make it limitless.

GM: Right. As a progressive, just as I don't want my tax dollars wasted on a bloated defense budget, I don't want my tax dollars paying for unnecessary angioplasties for bloated cheeseburger eaters. And I don't want my tax dollars to continue subsidizing the animal agriculture interests that are producing those low-cost cheeseburgers that are killing Americans. Stop subsidizing animal agriculture and let's see the real market cost of a cheeseburger, which may be fifteen dollars or more. Letting that cost rise to the market cost—something those free-market right-wingers should believe in—would do wonders for the state of American health.

PP: Here's my suggestion for Michael Moore, if he would ever listen to me. Michael, before you produce any more documentaries on health, I'm going to charge you with getting healthy. Your objective is to get thin and healthy. Once you go through the process of trying to do so—and you may well have already tried—and you find out how impossible it is to do by going through traditional medical channels, then do it like Bill Clinton did and try this whole food, plant-based diet. Go outside the system to find the answers to your health issues. Do that, and then you're going to produce a different kind of documentary, which will be well worth watching because you'll have some credibility on the subject.

GM: Lawrence O'Donnell, who as I mentioned deserves kudos for highlighting the absurdity of the mandate, nonetheless appears to agree with Michael Moore that the best system of health care would be Medicare for all. I was fortunate to have the chance recently to have a little private informal exchange with O'Donnell on the subject of health. Now, let me preface this by saying that the last thing in the world that I would want to do would be to attack Lawrence O'Donnell, who is a national treasure and as eloquent a spokesman for progressive values as anyone alive. But,

223

like Michael Moore and so many others on the left, he espouses ideas on public health policy that are reflexive expressions of an ideology that, despite its good intent, doesn't question common assumptions that our society makes on human health, many of which are profoundly wrong.

So I was delighted to have the chance to express to O'Donnell my frustration with media coverage of Obamacare over the last three years. I thought I made my case effectively, and here is the gist of what I said:

The media keeps referring to Obamacare as health reform when it is merely health insurance reform that affects health barely at all. Its essential flaw is its focus on insurance payments instead of health. I asked, with rhetorical flourish, would you rather have good health insurance or good health? The real problem in this country isn't the millions without health insurance; the real problems are obesity, diabetes, heart disease, and cancer. It's the food, stupid! Studies have shown that access to medical care has minimal effect on health outcomes; indeed, I noted, the third-leading cause of death in America is medical care. (O'Donnell disputed that assertion but I would point him to an op-ed by Dr. Sanjay Gupta in the *New York Times*, in which he estimated two hundred thousand iatrogenic deaths annually, which puts death by medical care in third place, as I contended.[9]) The one thing that truly has demonstrable effect on health outcomes is the food we eat. If we were to stop subsidizing the meat and dairy industry with farm subsidies, allowing the price of a cheeseburger to skyrocket, that would do more to improve human health than Obamacare ever could. Somebody in the media needs to let another voice into the debate besides the usual detractors and supporters of Obamacare. We need a voice like Dr. McDougall's that would make the case that we'll never solve the problem unless we change the food.

And I rested my argument, rather proud of myself.

PP: Was he left speechless?

GM: Actually, no. There's a reason Lawrence O'Donnell has risen as far as he has. He's a very persuasive guy. He dismissed my arguments like he was swatting so many flies and then moved on to his next interlocutor. First, he said, give up on the fantasy that we'll ever end farm subsidies. Second, he said, I simply was not allowing for human fallibility. Ice cream, he said, is delicious. He repeated that statement over and over, with increasing emphasis. "Ice cream is delicious. People will always eat ice cream because ice cream is DE-LIC-IOUS! That's never going to change. Human beings are fallible and, being fallible, will always eat ice cream because ICE CREAM IS DE-LIC-IOUS!" I was wasting my breath with all my impossibly severe ideas about eating.

I walked away deflated. Here I thought I had made several powerful arguments for why we needed to change the debate about health in this country, and yet I had made a rookie error, failing to factor in the extraordinary deliciousness of ice cream. I didn't know whether to keep fighting for the plant-based cause, or just chuck it all and head to Baskin-Robbins.

PP: Here's what O'Donnell is not taking into account. The American public is not given the opportunity to make an informed decision. Your cholesterol is 220, so your doctor says, "You know, your cholesterol is getting up there. We're going to need to put you on a statin drug." So he puts you on Lipitor and your cholesterol comes down. You get this false sense of security that things are better because you were never really told the whole story about your cholesterol. That sense of security ends with a heart attack. Now let's replay this conversation the way it should happen. You go to your doctor and your cholesterol is 220 and your doctor says, "Here are our choices. We can use Lipitor, and it'll reduce your risk of dying of a heart attack by about 1.8 percent. I want to read to you the list of side effects of the drug very briefly; it's just six or seven pages long. So you can take this drug, or I can show you how to eat a diet that will work faster than the drug and will reduce your risk of dying of a heart attack almost entirely. You'll also reduce your risk of dying from cancer, diabetes, and other diseases. And there are no side effects. Now, which would you like to do? I can either write the prescription right now, or I can teach you how to eat this diet."

I believe that most people, when presented with those alternatives, would at least take a look at this diet. I've worked with all kinds of people: blue-collar workers, white-collar workers, people who make $400,000 a year, people who make $20,000 a year. They don't all jump at the chance to change their diet, but a heck of a lot of them want to do it when presented with that kind of information. I think the public should be insulted by the mind-set that presumes that it does not have the will or the intelligence to make a change for its own good. What Lawrence O'Donnell is basically saying is that people are so stupid and weak that we might as well not even tell them about the ideal human diet because they'd rather eat ice cream and lose their limbs to diabetes than make the effort to clean up their diet.

GM: I think he's saying that people know that ice cream isn't a health food, but they eat it anyway because they are fallible creatures.

PP: No, they don't know. They're misled a hundred different ways. They're eating fat-free ice cream. They're told that dairy products provide calcium to strengthen their bones. They're told that chocolate is a superfood and that nuts are indispensable for brain function. And they're taught that they can't affect their health or their weight very much in any case because it's all in the genes. They look to the Academy of Nutrition and Dietetics for dietary advice and they're told that there's room for everything, including ice cream, in a healthy diet. They think that because they buy extra virgin olive oil, fat-free dairy products, and imported organic cheese, they're doing great. Lawrence O'Donnell was basically implying that 160 million Americans with degenerative disease are well aware that their current treatments don't work and that they can instead eat themselves out of disease, but they've just chosen not to do so because they love ice cream. Well, that's not been my experience. I find it unfathomable that people would care so little about themselves that, in spite of being well aware of how to regain their health, they just wouldn't want to make the effort. I don't believe that's the case at all.

I'll tell you what my experience has been, not with one or two people but with many thousands of people. When they understand the truth about what is making them sick, many act on it. They are willing to change their diets not just a little bit, but entirely. And the diet they adopt is full of foods that, to the palates they cultivate, are every bit as delicious as ice cream once was to them, when their palates responded only to sugar and fat. And, incidentally, once in a while on special occasions, they may still indulge in some delicious non-dairy ice cream. But they know that there's no reason to ever again touch dairy or the foods that have made them fat and sick.

This is the way our public health crisis ends. The government isn't going to do it. People have to do it. They have to take their health into their own hands. The job of the medical community is to give people the knowledge upon which they can act. If the medical community continues to fail in that responsibility, we in the plant-based foods movement will pick up the slack. We will get the word out in books, in films like *Forks Over Knives*, on the Internet, through educational ventures like The Wellness Forum, person-to-person, and in any other way we can. We will treat people with respect by giving them the knowledge upon which they will act to save their own lives and to save the country from a fiscal nightmare. I firmly believe that people can do this, and that's not blind optimism on my part. I see it happen every day.

GM: Pam, it's been a pleasure chatting with you, but I've got to go home and stay up late and type all of this up.

PP: Have a cup of coffee.

NOTES

. . . .

CHAPTER ONE

1 "India reworks obesity guidelines, BMI lowered," iGovernment, November 26, 2008, www.igovernment.in/site/India-reworks-obesity -guidelines-BMI-lowered/.
2 K. Trakas, K. Lawrence, and N. Shear, "Utilization of health care resources by obese Canadians," *Canadian Medical Association Journal*, 160, no. 10 (May 18, 1999): 1457–62.
3 "F as in Fat: How Obesity Threatens America's Future," Trust for America's Health, last modified September 2012, www.healthyamericans .org/assets/files/TFAH2012FasInFat18.pdf.
4 "Adult Obesity Facts," Centers for Disease Control, www.cdc.gov /obesity/data/adult.html.
5 H. Vorster, "Fructose and Blood Cholesterol," *American Journal of Clinical Nutrition* 57, no. 1 (January 1993): 89, www.ajcn.org /content/57/1/89.2.full.pdf.
6 D. Farlow, X. Xu, and T. Veenstra, "Quantitative measurement of endogenous estrogen metabolites, risk-factors for development of breast cancer, in commercial milk products by LC–MS/MS," *Journal of Chromatography B* 877, no. 13 (2009): doi:10.1016/j .jchromb.2009.01.032.
7 F. Crowe, T.J. Key, N.E. Allen, et al., "The association between diet and serum concentrations of IGF-I, IGFBP-1, IGFBP-2, and IGFBP-3 in the European Prospective Investigation into Cancer and Nutrition," *Cancer Epidemiology, Biomarkers & Prevention* 18, no. 5 (2009): 1333–40.

8   R. Heaney, D.A. McCarron, B. Dawson-Hughes, et al., "Dietary changes favorably affect bone remodeling in older adults," *Journal of the American Dietetic Association* 99, no. 10 (October 1999): 1228–33.

9   J. Chan , M.J. Stampfer, J. Ma, et al., "Insulin-like growth factor-1 (IGF-1) and IGF binding protein3 as predictors of advanced stage prostate cancer," *Journal of the National Cancer Institute* 94, no. 14 (July 17, 2002): 1099–1106.

CHAPTER TWO

1   R. Prentice, B. Caan, R.T. Chlebowski, et al., "Low-fat dietary pattern and risk of invasive breast cancer," *Journal of the American Medical Association* 295, no. 6 (February 8, 2006): 629–42.

2   D. Hegsted, "Minimum protein requirements of adults," *American Journal of Clinical Nutrition* 21, no. 5 (May 1968): 352–57.

3   A. Prentice, "Constituents of Breast Milk," United Nations University, *Food and Nutrition Bulletin* 17, no. 4 (December 1996): http://archive .unu.edu/unupress/food/8F174e/8F174E04.htm.

4   T. C. Campbell and T.M. Campbell II, *The China Study* (Dallas: Ben-Bella Books, 2004).

5   R.H. Chittenden, *Physiological economy in nutrition, with special reference to the minimal protein requirement of the healthy man. An experimental study* (New York: Frederick A. Stokes Co., 1907), 24-33, 255.

6   Ibid., 327.

7   Howard Lyman and Glen Merzer, *Mad Cowboy* (New York: Scribner, 1998), 147.

8   "Livestock's Long Shadow," Food and Agriculture Organization of the United Nations, last modified 2006, www.fao.org/docrep/010 /a0701e/a0701e00.HTM.

9   J. Chavarro, J.W. Rich-Edwards, B.A. Rosner, and W.C. Willet, "Diet and lifestyle in the prevention of ovulatory disorder infertility," *Obstetrics & Gynecology* 110, no. 5 (November 2007): 1050–58.

10 J. Chavarro et al., "Protein intake and ovulatory infertility," *American Journal of Obstetrics & Gynecology* 198, no. 2 (February 2008): 210.e-1-210.e-7.

11 J. Chavarro et al., "A prospective study of dairy foods intake and anovulatory infertility," *Human Reproduction* 22 no. 5 (May 2007): 1340–47.

CHAPTER THREE

1   J. Karjalainen, J.M. Martin, M. Knip, et al., "A bovine albumin peptide as a possible trigger of insulin-dependent diabetes mellitus," *New England Journal of Medicine* 327 (1992): 302–7.

2   H. Akerblom and M. Knip, "Putative environmental factors and Type 1 diabetes," *Diabetes/Metabolism Research and Reviews* 14 (1998): 31–67.

3   E. Savilahti, H.K. Akerblom, V.M. Tainio, and S. Koskimies, "Children with newly diagnosed insulin dependent diabetes mellitus have increased levels of cow's milk antibodies," *Diabetes Research and Clinical Practice* 7, no. 3 (March 1988): 137–40.

4   W. Oddy, P.G. Holt, P.D. Sly, et al., "Association between breast feeding and asthma in 6 year old children: findings of a prospective birth cohort study," *BMJ* 319 (September 25, 1999): 815.

5   S. Koletzko, P. Sherman, M. Corey, A. Giffiths, and C. Smith, "Role of infant feeding practices in development of Crohn's disease in childhood," *BMJ* 298 (June 17, 1989): 1617–18.

6   A. Austin, A. Santhanam, and Z. Katusic, "Endothelial nitric oxide modulates expression and processing of amyloid precursor protein," *Circulation Research* 107 (2010): 1498–1502.

7   N. Shepardson, G. Shankar, and D. Selkoe, "Cholesterol level and statin use in Alzheimer disease: II. Review of human trials and recommendations," *Archives of Neurology & Psychiatry* 68, no. 11 (November 2011): 1385–92, doi:10.1001/archneurol.2011.242.

8   A. Mandell, M. Alexander, and S. Carpenter, "Creutzfeldt-Jakob disease presenting as isolated aphasia," *Neurology* 39, no. 1 (January 1989): 55–58.

9   M. Morris, D.A. Evans, J.L. Bienias, et al., "Dietary fats and the risk of incident Alzheimer disease," *Archives of Neurology & Psychiatry* 60, no. 2 (February 2003): 194–200.

10   A. Neviaser, J.M. Lane, B.A. Lenart, F. Edobor-Osula, and D.G. Lorich, "Low-energy femoral shaft fractures associated with alendronate use," *Journal of Orthopaedic Trauma* 22 (2008): 346–50.

11   P. Sedghizadeh, K. Stanley, M. Caligiuri, et al., "Oral bisphosphonate use and the prevalence of osteonecrosis of the jaw: an institutional inquiry," *Journal of the American Dental Association* 140, no. 1 (January 2009): 61–66.

12   R. Moynihan, I. Heath, and D. Henry, "Selling sickness: the pharmaceutical industry and disease mongering," *BMJ* 324 (2002): 886–91.

13   D. Marshall, O. Johnell, and H. Wedel, "Meta-analysis of how well measures of bone mineral density predict occurrence of osteoporotic fractures," *BMJ* 312 (May 18, 1996): 1254–59.

14   D. Hegsted, "Calcium and Osteoporosis," *Journal of Nutrition* 116 (July 15, 1986): 2316–19.

15   A. Wachsman and D. Bernstein, "Diet and Osteoporosis," *Lancet* 291, no. 7549 (May 4, 1968): 958–59.

16   U. Barzel and L. Massey, "Excess dietary protein can adversely affect bone," *Journal of Nutrition* 128, no. 6 (June 1998): 1051–53

17   S. Margen, J.Y. Chu, N.A. Kaufmann, and D.H. Calloway, "Studies in calcium metabolism. I. The calciuretic effect of dietary protein," *American Journal of Clinical Nutrition* 27 (June 1974): 584–89

18   M. Hegsted , S.A. Schuette, M.B. Zemel, and H.M. Linkswiler, "Urinary calcium and calcium balance in young men as affected by level

of protein and phosphorus intake," *Journal of Nutrition* 111 (1981): 553–62.

[19] Amy Joy Lanou and Michael Castleman, *Building Bone Vitality* (New York: McGraw-Hill, 2009), 111–14.

[20] Food and Agriculture Organization of the United Nations, *The State of Food and Agriculture – 1948* (Washington, DC, September 1948).

[21] R. Swank, O. Lerstad, A. Stromm, and J. Backer, "Multiple sclerosis in rural Norway: its geographic and occupational incidence in relation to nutrition," *New England Journal of Medicine*, 246 (May 8, 1952): 721–28.

[22] R. Swank and B. Dugan, "Effect of low saturated fat diet in early and late cases of multiple sclerosis," *Lancet* 336, no. 8706 (July 7, 1990): 37–39.

[23] Ibid.

[24] R. Swank, "Treatment of multiple sclerosis with low fat diet," *Archives of Neurology & Psychiatry* 69, no. 1 (1953): 91.

[25] R. Swank and R. Bourdillon, "Multiple sclerosis: assessment of treatment with a modified low-fat diet," *Journal of Nervous and Mental Disease* 131, no. 6 (December 1960): 468–88.

[26] R. Swank, "Multiple sclerosis: twenty years on low-fat diet," *Archives of Neurology* 23 (November 1970): 460–74.

[27] H. Sampson, "Food allergy. Part 1: immunopathogenesis and clinical disorders," *Journal of Allergy and Clinical Immunology* 103, no. 5 (May 1999): 717–28.

[28] A. Host, "Frequency of cow's milk allergy in childhood," *Annals of Allergy, Asthma and Immunology* 89, no. 6 Suppl 1 (December 2002): 33–37.

[29] P. Potter, M. Klein, and E. Weinberg, "Hydration in severe acute asthma," *Archives of Disease in Childhood* 66 (1991): 216–19, doi:10.1136/adc.66.2.216.

[30] M. Gunnbjörnsdóttir, E. Omenaas, T. Gíslason, et al., on behalf of the RHINE study group, "Obesity and nocturnal gastro-oesophageal reflux are related to onset of asthma and respiratory symptoms," *European Respiratory Journal* 24 (2004): 116–21.

[31] A. Barbas, T.E. Downing, K.R. Balsara, et al., "Chronic aspiration shifts the immune response from Th1 to Th2 in a murine model of asthma," *European Journal of Clinical Investigation* 38, no. 8 (July 17, 2008): 596–602.

[32] J. Lagergren, Y. Weimin, and A. Ekbom, "Intestinal cancer after cholecystectomy: is bile involved in carcinogenesis?" *Gastroenterology* 121, no. 3 (September 2001): 542–47.

[33] M. Dominguez , E.K. Costello, M. Contreras, et al., "Delivery mode shapes the acquisition and structure of the initial microbiota across multiple body habitats in newborns," *Proceedings of the National Academy of Sciences* 107, no. 26 (June 29, 2010): 11971–75.

[34] L. Morelli, "Postnatal development of intestinal microflora as

influenced by infant nutrition," *Journal of Nutrition* 138 (2008): 1791S–95S.

35 S. Zar, D. Kumar, and M. Benson, "Review article: food hypersensitivity and irritable bowel syndrome," *Alimentary Pharmacology & Therapeutics* 15 (2001): 439–49.

36 K. Heaton, J. Thornton, and P. Emmett, "Treatment of Crohn's disease with an unrefined carbohydrate, fibre-rich diet," *BMJ* 2 (1979): 764–66.

37 Shannon Brownlee, *Overtreated: Why Too Much Medicine Is Making Us Sicker and Poorer* (New York: Bloomsbury, 2008).

38 B. Starfield, "Is U.S. health really the best in the world?" *Journal of the American Medical Association* 284, no. 4 (July 26, 2000): 483–85, doi:10-1001/pubs.JAMA-ISSN-0098-7484-284-4-jco00061.

39 N. Allen, C. Sauvaget, and A. Roddam, "A prospective study of diet and prostate cancer in Japanese men," *Cancer Causes & Control* 15 (2004): 911–20.

40 P. Barter, M. Caulfield, M. Eriksson, et al., "Effects of torcetrapib in patients at high risk for coronary events," *New England Journal of Medicine* 357 (November 22, 2007): 2109–22.

41 W. Connor, M.T. Cerqueira, R.W. Connor, et al., "The plasma lipids, lipoproteins, and diet of the Tarahumara Indians of Mexico," *American Journal of Clinical Nutrition* 31 (July 1978): 1131–42.

42 J. Bernstein, "The role of IgE-mediated hypersensitivity in the development of otitis media with effusion," *Otolaryngologic Clinics of North America* 25, no. 1 (February 1992): 197–211.

43 H. Juntti, S. Tikkanen, J. Kokkonen, O.P. Alho, and A. Niinimäki, "Cow's milk allergy is associated with recurrent otitis media during childhood," *Acta Oto-Laryngologica* 119, no. 8 (1999): 867–73.

44 D. Malosse and H. Perron, "Correlation analysis between bovine populations, other farm animals, house pets, and multiple sclerosis prevalence," *Neuroepidemiology* 12, no. 1 (1993): 15–27.

45 J. Chan and E. Giovannucci, "Dairy products, calcium and vitamin D and risk of prostate cancer," *Epidemiologic Reviews* 23, no. 1 (2001): 87–92.

46 D. Feskanich, W.C. Willet, M.J. Stampfer, and G.A. Colditz, "Milk, dietary calcium, and bone fractures in women: a 12-year prospective study," *American Journal of Public Health* 87, no. 6 (June 1997): 992–97.

47 J. Karjalainen et al., "Bovine albumin peptide as a possibe trigger," 302–7.

48 H. Akerblom and M. Knip, "Putative environmental factors and Type 1 diabetes," *Diabetes/Metabolism Reviews* 14 (1998): 31–67.

49 C. Verge, N.J. Howard, L. Irwig, et al., "Environmental factors in childhood IDDM," *Diabetes Care* 17, no. 12 (December 1994): 1381–9.

50 L. Appel, N.J. Howard, L. Irwig, et al., "A clinical trial of the effects of dietary patterns on blood pressure," *New England Journal of Medicine* 336 (April 17, 1997): 1117–24.

51 H. Cohen, S. Hailpern, J. Fang, and M.H. Alderman, "Sodium intake and mortality in the NHANES II follow-up study," *American Journal of Medicine* 119, no. 3 (March 2006): 275.e.7-14.

52 M. Alderman, "Reducing dietary sodium: the case for caution," *Journal of the American Medical Association* 303, no. 5 (February 3, 2010): 448–49.

53 A. Bernstein and W. Willett, "Trends in 24-h urinary sodium excretion in the United States, 1957–2003: a systematic review," *American Journal of Clinical Nutrition* 92 (2010): 1172–80.

54 "Global Status Report on Noncommunicable Diseases 2010," World Health Organization, www.who.int/nmh/publications/ncd_report_full_en.pdf.

55 A. Buitrago-Lopez, J. Sanderson, L. Johnson, et al., "Chocolate consumption and cardiometabolic disorders: systematic review and meta-analysis," *BMJ* 343 (August 29, 2011): d4488, doi:10.1136/bmj.d4488.

CHAPTER FIVE

1 Roni Caryn Rabin, "Childhood Obesity and School Lunches," *New York Times*, February 8, 2011, D6.

2 "Dietary Guidelines: Urgent Prescription for an Unhealthy Public, Says American Dietetic Association," Academy of Nutrition and Dietetics (formerly American Dietetic Association), Media Room, www.eatright.org/Media/content.aspx?id=6442462223.

3 Academy of Nutrition and Deitetics. *Who Are the Academy's Corporate Sponsors?* www.eatright.org/corporatesponsors/ (accessed November 7, 2012).

4 T.C. Campbell and T.M. Campbell II, *The China Study* (Dallas: BenBella Books, 2004).

5 "Fecal Contamination in Retail Chicken Products," Physicians Committee for Responsible Medicine, April 2012, www.pcrm.org/health/reports/fecal-contamination-in-retail-chicken-products.

6 "U.S. per Capita Meat Consumption 1950–2007," USDA, Economic Research Service, https://d3n8a8pro7vhmx.cloudfront.net/foodday/pages/24/attachments/original/1342127278/High-Meat_Diet_Consequences.pdf?1342127278.

7 Peter Breggin and David Cohen, *Your Drug May Be Your Problem* (Da Capo Press, 1999): 125–26, 128, 133.

8 Statement by David J. Graham, U.S. Senate Committee on Finance, *Hearing on Vioxx*, November 18, 2004 (accessed November 7, 2012).

9 Thomas M. Burton and Jennifer Dooren, "Key FDA Approval Yanked for Avastin," *Wall Street Journal*, November 19, 2011.

10 "Feel Good About Loving Beef," Beef Checkoff, www.beefitswhatsfordinner.com/beefhealth.aspx.

11 A. Ault and J. Bradbury, "Experts argue about tamoxifen prevention trial," *Lancet* 351, no. 9109 (April 11, 1998): 1107.

12 N. Barnard, L. Scherwitz, and D. Ornish, "Adherence and acceptability of a low-fat, vegetarian diet among patients with cardiac disease," *Journal of Cardiopulmonary Rehabilitation and Prevention* 12, no. 6 (November 1992): 383-453.

13 N.D. Barnard, L. Gloede, J. Cohen, et al., "A low-fat vegan diet elicits greater macronutrient changes, but is comparable in adherence and acceptability, compared with a more conventional diabetes diet among individuals with Type 2 diabetes," *Journal of the American Dietetic Association* 109, no. 2 (February 2009): 263–72.

CHAPTER SIX

1 Sharon Begley, "One Word Can Save Your Life: No!" *Newsweek*, August 14, 2011.

2 R.S. Hayward, E.P. Steinberg, D.E. Ford, M.F. Roizen, and K.W. Roach, "Preventive care guidelines: 1991," *Annals of Internal Medicine* 114, no. 9 (May 1, 1991): 758–83.

3 J. Smith, J. Green, A. Berrington de Gonzalz, et al., "Cervical cancer and the use of hormonal contraceptives: a systemic review," *Lancet* 361, no. 9364 (April 5, 2003): 1159–67.

4 O. Olsen and P. Gotzsche, "Cochrane review on screening for breast cancer with mammography," *Lancet* 358, no. 9290 (October 20, 2001): 1340–42.

5 Peter Gotzsche, *Mammography Screening: Truth Lies and Controversy* (London: Radcliffe Publishing, 2012).

6 K. Jorgensen, P. Zahl, and P. Gotzsche, "Breast cancer mortality in organised mammography screening in Denmark: comparative study," *BMJ* 340 (March 24, 2010): c1241, doi:10.1136/bmj.c1241.

7 A. Berrington de Gonzalez, C.D. Berg, K. Visvanathan, and M. Robson, "Estimated risk of radiation-induced breast cancer from mammographic screening for young BRCA mutation carriers," *Journal of the National Cancer Institute* 101 (2009): 205–9, doi:10.1093/jnci/djn440.

8 C. Schmidt, "CT scans: balancing health risks and medical benefits," *Environmental Health Perspectives* 120, no. 3 (March 1, 2012): doi: a118–a121, doi:10.1289/ehp.120-a118.

9 R. Smith-Bindman, W. Hosmer, V.A. Feldstein, J.J. Deeks, and J.D. Goldberg, "Second-trimester ultrasound to detect fetuses with Down syndrome: a meta-analysis," *Journal of the American Medical Association* 285, no. 8 (2001): 1044–55.

10 H. Gilbert Welch, Lisa M. Schwartz, and Steven Woloshin, *Overdiagnosed* (Boston: Beacon Press, 2011), 138–40.

11 A. Neugut and B. Lebwohl, "Colonoscopy vs sigmoidoscopy screening: getting it right," *Journal of the American Medical Association* 304, no. 4 (2010): 461–62, doi:10.1001/jama.2010.1001.

12 Richard Ablin, "The Great Prostate Mistake," *New York Times*, March 9, 2012.

13 "Screening for Prostate Cancer: U.S. Preventive Services Task Force Recommendation Statement," U.S. Preventive Services Task Force, last modified May 2012, www.uspreventiveservicestaskforce.org/prostate cancerscreening/prostatefinalrs2.htm.

14 A. Kavanagh, G. Santow, and H. Mitchell, "Consequences of current patterns of pap smear and colposcopy use," *Journal of Medical Screening* 3, no. 1 (1996): 29–34.

15 "Ob-Gyns Recommend Women Wait 3 to 5 Years Between PAP Tests," The American Congress of Obstetricians and Gynecologists, news release, October 22, 2012, http://www.acog.org/About_ACOG /News_Room/News_Releases/2012/.

16 Ryan Janslow, "Doctors unveil 'Choosing Wisely' campaign to cut unnecessary medical tests," CBSNews.com, April 4, 2012, www .cbsnews.com/8301-504763_162-57409204-10391704/doctors-unveil -choosing-wisely-campaign-to-cut-unnecessary-medical-tests.

17 "Five Things Physicians and Patients Should Question," http://choosing wisely.org.

18 Peter Breggin, *Your Drug May Be Your Problem* (Boston: Da Capo Press, 1999), 72–73.

19 J. Gotto and M. Rapaport, "Treatment Options in Treatment-Resistant Depression," *Primary Psychiatry* 12, no. 2 (2005): 42–50, www.psychweekly.com/aspx/article/ArticleDetail.aspx?articleid=53.

CHAPTER SEVEN

1 M. Pereira, D.R. Jacobs Jr., L. Van Horn, et al., "Dairy consumption, obesity, and the insulin resistance syndrome in young adults: The CARDIA study," *Journal of the American Medical Association* 287, no. 16 (2002): 2081–89.

2 Caldwell B. Esselstyn Jr., *Prevent and Reverse Heart Disease* (New York: Penguin, 2007), 48.

3 Bill Moyers, *Healing and The Mind* (New York: Doubleday, 1993), 89.

4 W. Haenszel and M. Kurihara, "Studies of Japanese migrants: mortality from cancer and other disease among Japanese and the United States," *Journal of the National Cancer Institute* 40, no. 1 (1968): 43–68, doi:10.1093/jnci/40.1.43.

5 B. Armstrong and R. Doll, "Environmental factors and cancer incidence and mortality in different countries, with special reference to dietary practices," *International Journal of Cancer* 15 (1975): 617–31.

6 W. Lands, T. Hamazakim K. Yamazaki, et al., "Changing dietary patterns," *American Journal of Clinical Nutrition* 51 (1990): 991–93.

7 W. Haenszel and M. Kurihara, "Studies of Japanese migrants: mortality from cancer and other diseases among Japanese in the United

States," *Journal of the National Cancer Institute* 40, no. 1 (1968): 43–68, doi: 10.1093/jnci/40.1.43.

8 L.O. Schulz, P.H. Bennett, E. Ravussin, et al., "Effects of traditional and western environments on prevalence of type 2 diabetes in Pima Indians in Mexico and the U.S.," *Diabetes Care* 29, no. 8 (August 2006): 1866–71, doi:10.2337/dc06-0138.

9 L. Hooper, R.L. Thompson, R.A. Harrison, et al., "Risks and benefits of Omega 3 fats for mortality, cardiovascular disease, and cancer: systematic review," *BMJ* 332, no. 7544 (April 1, 2006): 752–60, doi:10.1136/bmj.38755.366331.2F.

10 G. Bjelakovic, D. Nikolova, L.L. Gluud, R.G. Simonetti, and C. Gluud, "Antioxidant supplements for prevention of mortality in healthy participants and patients with various diseases," *Cochrane Database of Systematic Reviews 2008*, Issue 2, Art. No.: CD007176, doi:10.1002/14651858.CD007176.pub2.

11 H. Lange, H. Surypranata, G. De Luca, et al., "Folate therapy and in-stent restenosis after coronary stenting," *New England Journal of Medicine* 26, no. 350 (June 24, 2004): 2673–81.

12 D. Wu and S.N. Mevdani, "n-3 polyunsaturated fatty acids and im-mune function," *Proceedings of the Nutrition Society* 57, no. 4 (November 1998): 503–9.

13 D. Blankenhorn, R.L. Johnson, W.J. Mack, H.A. el Zein, and L.I. Vailas, "The influence of diet on the appearance of new lesions in human coronary arteries," *Journal of the American Medical Association* 263, no. 12 (March 23, 1990): 1646–52.

14 N. Barnard et al., "Adherence and Acceptability of a Low-Fat Vegetarian Diet," 383-453; N. Barnard, L. Gloede, J. Cohen, et al., "A low-fat vegan diet and a conventional diabetes diet in the treatment of type 2 diabetes: a randomized, controlled, 74-wk clinical trial," *American Journal of Clinical Nutrition* 89, no. 5 (May 2009): 1588S-1596S.

15 N. Barnard et al., "Vegan diet elicits greater macronutrient changes," 263–72.

16 J.W. Anderson, "Dietary fiber in nutrition management of diabetes," in *Dietary Fiber: Basic and Clinical Aspects*, ed. G. V. Vahouny, and D. Kritchevsky (New York: Plenum Press, 1986), 343–60.

17 P. Peduzzi, A. Kamina, and K. Detre, for The VA Coronary Artery Bypass Surgery Cooperative Study Group, Twenty-two-year follow-up in the VA Cooperative Study of Coronary Artery Bypass Surgery for Stable Angina," *American Journal of Cardiology* 81 (1998): 1393–99.

18 "Long-term results of prospective randomised study of coronary artery bypass surgery in stable angina pectoris," European Coronary Surgery Study Group, *Lancet* 2, no. 8309 (November 27, 1982): 1173–80.

19 B.R. Chaitman, T.J. Ryan, R.A. Kronmal, et al., "Coronary Artery Surgery Study (CASS): comparability of 10 year survival in random-ized and randomizable patients," *Journal of the American College of Cardiology* 16, no. 5 (November 1990): 1071–78.

20   D. Cohen, J. Carozza, and D. Baim, "Aggressive lipid-lowering therapy compared with angioplasty in stable coronary artery disease," *New England Journal of Medicine* 341 (December 9, 1999): 1853–55, doi:10.1056/NEJM199912093412415.

21   "Coronary Angioplasty and Stenting," University of Michigan Health System Cardiac Surgery, www.med.umich.edu/cardiac-surgery/patient/adult/adultcandt/coronary_angioplasty.shtml.

22   "Bypass Surgery and Memory," The Harvard Medical School Family Health Guide, www.health.harvard.edu/fhg/updates/update0206c.shtml.

23   "Crestor Highlights of Prescribing Information," AstraZeneca, fact sheet, www1.astrazeneca-us.com/pi/crestor.pdf.

CHAPTER EIGHT

1   David Squires, "Explaining High Health Care Spending in the United States: An International Comparison of Supply, Utilization, Prices, and Quality," The Commonwealth Fund, April 2012, http://www.commonwealthfund.org/~/media/Files/Publications/Issue%20Brief/2012/May/1595_Squires_explaining_high_hlt_care_spending_intl_brief.pdf.

2   "The Healthy School Meals Act of 2010 (Rep. Jared Polis, CO)" fact sheet, http://static.usnews.com/documents/whispers/Healthy_School_Meals_Act_of_2010_Fact_Sheet.pdf.

3   Richard Rushfield, "Trapped in Men's Central Jail," *L.A. Weekly*, April 5, 2012, http://digitalissue.laweekly.com/display_article.php?id=1025278.

4   "Bay Point School for Boys," The Food Studies Institute, www.foodstudies.org/index.php?option=com_content&view=article&id=19&Itemid=27.

5   B. Scott , F.C. Seifert, R. Grimson, and P.S.A. Glass, "Octogenarians undergoing coronary artery bypass graft surgery: resource utilization, postoperative mortality and morbidity," *Journal of Cardiothoracic and Vascular Anesthesia* 19, no. 5 (October 2005): 583–88.

6   V.L. Ernster, "Mammography screening for women age 40 through 49: a guidelines saga and a clarion call for informed decision making," *American Journal of Public Health* 87, no. 7 (1997): 1103–6.

7   "Animals Killed for Food in the U.S. Increases in 2010," blog post, OneGreenPlanet.org, October 21, 2011, www.onegreenplanet.org/news/animals-killed-for-food-in-the-u-s-increases-in-2010.

8   Alice Park, "NYC's Trans Fat Ban Worked: Fast-Food Diners Are Eating Healthier," *Time*, July 17, 2012, http://healthland.time.com/2012/07/17/nycs-trans-fat-ban-worked-fast-food-diners-are-eating-healthier.

9   Dr. Sanjay Gupta, "More Treatment, More Mistakes," *New York Times*, July 31, 2012, www.nytimes.com/2012/08/01/opinion/more-treatment-more-mistakes.html.

ABOUT THE AUTHORS

. . . .

DR. PAMELA A. POPPER, PH.D., N.D.

D r. Pam Popper is a naturopath; an internationally recognized expert on nutrition, medicine, and health; and the executive director of The Wellness Forum. The company offers educational programs designed to assist individuals in changing their health outcomes through improved diet and lifestyle habits; to assist employers in reducing the costs of health insurance and medical care for employees; and to educate health care professionals about how to use diet and lifestyle for preventing, reversing, and stopping the progression of degenerative disease.

Dr. Popper serves on the Physicians' Steering Committee for the Physicians Committee for Responsible Medicine in Washington, D.C. She is also one of the health care professionals involved in the famed Sacramento Food Bank Project, in which economically disadvantaged people were shown how to reverse their diseases and eliminate medications with diet.

Dr. Popper is part of Dr. T. Colin Campbell's teaching team at eCornell, teaching part of a certification course on plant-based nutrition. She has been featured in many widely distributed documentaries, including *Processed People*, *Making a Killing*, and *Forks Over Knives*, which opened in theaters in May 2011. She is one of the coauthors of the *Forks Over Knives* companion book, which is on the *New York Times* best-seller list.

GLEN MERZER

Glen Merzer is coauthor with Howard Lyman of *Mad Cowboy*, and with Howard Lyman and Joanna Samorow-Merzer of *No More Bull!* He is also coauthor of Chef AJ's *Unprocessed*, and of the forthcoming *Better Than Vegan*, with Chef Del Sroufe. He is also a playwright and screenwriter, with three plays published by Samuel French, Inc. He has been a vegetarian for almost forty years, and a vegan for almost twenty.